Aphasia
in Clinical Practice

British Library Cataloguing in Publication Data
A catalogue record for this book is available from the British Library
Book and cover design: Jim Wilkie. Cover image by Cassette Bleue
(used under license from Shutterstock.com)

Index compiled by Terence Halliday

Printed and bound by CPI Group (UK) Ltd, Croydon, CR0 4YY

Aphasia
in Clinical Practice

Dee Webster (Editor)

J&R Press Ltd

For Seth & Ezra

Contents

About the contributors

Mary Agresta Spouse of individual with aphasia & strong advocate for people with aphasia.

Danny Dichiera Individual with aphasia and member of Aphasia SA (formerly Talkback Association Inc.).

Deborah Hersh, PhD, is Professor of Speech Pathology at Curtin University in Western Australia. She has over 30 years of clinical, teaching and research experience, is a Fellow of Speech Pathology Australia and is currently Chairperson of the Australian Aphasia Association. Her research uses a variety of qualitative approaches and includes a focus on person-centred practice, advocacy, patient and public involvement in research, culturally secure services for Aboriginal Australians, and therapeutic relationships. In particular, she has explored the experiences of people with aphasia and their families in relation to assessment, goal setting, discharge, and community aphasia groups.

Dr Mark Jayes Research Fellow in Communication Disability and Speech and Language Therapist Department of Health Professions Manchester Metropolitan University, UK.

Dr Helen Kelly Speech & Language Therapist and Lecturer, School of Clinical Therapies, University College Cork, County Cork, Republic of Ireland.

Dr Posy Knights Lead Clinical Psychologist for Stroke Nottinghamshire Healthcare NHS Foundation Trust, UK.

Dr Eirini Kontou Senior Research Fellow and Highly Specialist Clinical Psychologist in Stroke School of Medicine, Institute of Mental Health, University of Nottingham & Nottinghamshire Healthcare NHS Foundation Trust, UK.

Larry Masterson Founder, Different Strokes for Different Folks, County Donegal, Republic of Ireland.

Carol McGriskin Wife and Carer, Nottingham Stroke Research Forum Nottinghamshire, UK.

Peter McGriskin Stroke survivor and aphasia expert by experience. Nottinghamshire Aphasia Advisory Panel/Expert trainer with aphasia/ Nottingham Stroke Research Forum Nottinghamshire, UK.

Dr Sarah Northcott, Senior Lecturer, City, University of London, UK.

Eileen O'Riordan Aphasia expert, Aphasia Home Café, University College Cork, County Kerry, Republic of Ireland.

Philip Scott Aphasia expert; My Journey with Aphasia and Aphasia Home Café, University College Cork, County Cork, Republic of Ireland.

John Smejka Stroke survivor, Lincolnshire, UK.

Paula Smejka Family member, Lincolnshire, UK.

Dr Shirley Thomas Associate Professor in Rehabilitation Psychology School of Medicine, University of Nottingham, UK.

Jen Thomson Stroke Rehabilitation Speech and Language Therapist, Leeds Teaching Hospitals Trust, Leeds, UK.

Dee Webster University Teacher, Division of Human Communication Sciences, Health Sciences School, University of Sheffield, UK Highly Specialist Speech & Language Therapist, Nottinghamshire Healthcare NHS Foundation Trust, UK.

Tracey Wood Individual with aphasia and member of Aphasia WA.

About the Editor

Dee Webster is a Speech and Language Therapist specializing in stroke and aphasia. She works both in the NHS as a lead stroke clinician and also as a University Teacher at the University of Sheffield, UK. She is co-founder and Chair of the East Midlands and Yorkshire Aphasia Clinical Excellence Network and has previously been part of the British Aphasiology Society committee.

Dee's roles afford her the privilege of working alongside people with aphasia and their families, Speech and Language Therapy students, and both newly-qualified and more experienced clinicians. It is through these many conversations and interactions that the initial idea for this book was shaped, with a focus on aiming to represent and consider some of the key current clinical practices in aphasia from an authentic, real-word perspective.

This book brings together the voices and expertise of people with aphasia, researchers and clinicians across a range of topics which are pertinent to our clinical work with people with aphasia and their families.

1 "I just wanting talking to get better": Real-world perspectives on goal setting for aphasia rehabilitation

Deborah Hersh, Mary Agresta, Danny Dichiera and Tracey Wood

In their introduction to their book on goal setting in rehabilitation, Levack and Siegert (2015) explain how goal setting is usually approached in mainstream rehabilitation. Goals describe a "desired future state to be achieved by a person with a disability as a result of rehabilitation activities" (p.13). With their focus on function, Levack and Siegert suggest clinicians tend to orientate patients to activities of daily living or key life roles. Goals are usually formulated by the rehabilitation team with patients and families and are often influenced by recent assessment results and information gathered about the person and their background. Goals are typically presented as long-term (for the duration of rehabilitation, and perhaps beyond) with short-term goals identified as intermediary steps to get there. They are then phrased in a standard way to fit a SMART framework (Schut & Stam, 1994): that goals are *specific, measurable, achievable, realistic/relevant* and *timebound*. This all sounds straightforward, but of course it is not. As Levack et al. (2015) write:

> Goal setting is an inherently attractive concept, appearing deceptively simple at first and belying the complex relationships that exist between goals, personality, motivation, mood, self-regulation and other types of cognition. (p.21)

Goal setting encounters are not context-free. For example, rehabilitation clinicians may privilege goals they perceive to follow the funding or systemic expectations of their workplace, such as those with shorter timeframes which appear achievable, or that focus on physical function and help towards discharge (Levack, Dean, Siegert, & McPherson, 2011). Goal setting may also be shaped by health professionals' styles of interaction and orientated towards biomedical or behavioural goals (Franklin et al., 2019). In the context of stroke, research studies have found similar patterns in the way health professionals run goal setting (Barnard, Cruice, & Playford, 2010; Leach, Cornwell, Fleming, & Haines, 2010; Parry, 2004). Systematic reviews of the extensive body of research on goal setting in stroke rehabilitation (Levack, Weatherall, et al., 2015; Rosewilliam, Roskell, & Pandyan, 2011; Sugavanam, Mead, Bulley, Donaghy, & van Wijck, 2013) suggest that despite aiming for collaboration and a patient-centred process, significant barriers remain to achieving this in practice. Sugavanam and colleagues (2013) noted that: "patients were often unclear regarding their role in the goal setting process and did not participate fully…" (p.187). Rosewilliam et al. (2011) highlighted how systems were "too structured with dominating formal assessments which restricted exploration of patients' preferences and potential" (p.509). Moreover, studies exploring experiences of stroke patients about their goal setting in post-acute rehabilitation have found patients think very differently to health professionals about goals, often choosing "vague or broadly worded goals" (Brown et al., 2014, p.1024) and focusing on their need to manage day by day, deal with uncertainty, and demonstrate progress. Alanko, Karhula, Kröger, Piirainen & Nikander (2019) also explored experiences of goal setting by running interviews with 20 people, 13 of whom were post stroke. This study suggested that goal setting was deeply entwined in notions of trust (in the system, health professionals, families and even themselves) and that people often found the process of goal setting confusing. Their ability to engage in the process was diminished by pain, feeling unwell and by the fear of being unable to predict their recovery and situation.

Unsurprisingly, the ability to manage collaborative goal setting is likely to be more difficult when people have aphasia after stroke, and there is now also a specific literature on this topic (Berg, Rise, Balandin, Armstrong, & Askim, 2016; Berg, Askim, Balandin, Armstrong, & Rise, 2017; Brown, Brady, Worrall, & Scobbie, 2021; Elston et al., 2021; Haley, Cunningham, Barry, & de Riesthal, 2019; Hersh, Worrall, Howe, Sherratt, & Davidson, 2012a; Hersh et al., 2012b; Howe et al., 2012; Rohde, Townley-O'Neill, Trendall, Worrall & Cornwell, 2012; Sherratt et al., 2011; Worrall et al., 2011). Considering people with aphasia have often been excluded from studies on goal setting in stroke more generally, for example, those mentioned above by Brown et al. (2014) and Alanko et al. (2019), this research focus is important. Haley et al. (2019) note the three most common reasons why collaborative goal setting with people with aphasia can be difficult: there is often a lack of time to build a sufficiently detailed picture of the client and a tendency to rely on assessment results to inform therapy direction; clients are perceived as passive and find it hard to explain what they want to do; and the aphasia itself impacts on the ability to engage productively. Goal setting with people with aphasia may be viewed by health professionals in the multidisciplinary stroke team as the responsibility of the speech pathologist, particularly where other team members do not feel sufficiently skilled to use supportive communication strategies as a way to make the process of goal setting accessible (Haley et al., 2019; Brown et al., 2020). This reduces the likelihood of a collaborative goal setting process emerging within all the various therapies offered by the stroke team.

In this chapter, we aim to explore goal setting for people with aphasia set against the complex context described above, but in three different ways. First, we do so collaboratively, co-authoring between a speech pathologist/researcher (Deborah), two people with aphasia (Danny and Tracey), and Danny's spouse, Mary. The collaboration drew on existing relationships through local aphasia organizations. All authors have chosen to use their real names, and all have contributed knowledge to the chapter content as specified in the Authorship Guide developed by the National Health and Medical Research Council (2019). The material for this chapter was gathered through discussions which Deborah recorded and transcribed. Deborah spoke to Mary and Danny together, and to Tracey individually. She then drafted the chapter and checked back, through further discussion, to validate agreement that each person's views were clearly conveyed. This collaboration has been helpful in bringing together different experiences to co-construct the chapter rather than following the common reporting of clients' perspectives separately from, or contrasting with, therapists' perspectives. Second, this chapter brings an opportunity to hear contextualized goal setting stories, particularly through Mary's voice on behalf of herself and Danny, and from Tracey in conversation with Deborah. Many publications reporting on client perspectives of goal setting take a thematic view across multiple study participants and illustrate with quotations which are decontextualized or removed from their broader narratives of recovery. We will show how goal setting can be appreciated when placed back in the bigger 'real world' picture for an individual by sharing stories – and we argue that this may help clinicians reflect and set goals with clients more effectively. Finally, we look at goal setting down the recovery track, a novel perspective because much of the research on this topic has focused on the acute and sub-acute rehabilitation phase. It is well known that aphasia recovery is a long process (Wray & Clarke, 2017), and that people may still receive therapy years after the stroke. However, goal setting issues in the longer term, and how goals adjust over time (Scobbie. Thomson, Pollock, & Evans, 2020), are highlighted less often. Here, we will show that the process of working out a mutually agreed therapy direction remains complex for people with chronic aphasia.

The chapter is organized by examining these three aspects through reference to the *SMARTER* goal setting framework (Hersh et al., 2012a), a way of conceptualizing and remembering important and overlapping features of the goal setting process. *SMARTER* is an acronym which stands for *Shared, Monitored, Accessible, Relevant, Transparent, Evolving* and *Relationship-Centred*. It was developed from a study which involved interviews with 132 people across Australia (Worrall et al., 2011) – 50 people with aphasia, 48 family members and 34 treating speech pathologists. As such, we have found it a useful framework to structure and bring together salient points from each of our perspectives. We use our stories and experiences to illustrate what goal setting looks like within real-world recovery journeys.

Real-world perspectives

Danny was a lawyer, keen footballer and cricketer, who also loved amateur dramatics and performing in the annual fringe festival. Following a visit to a chiropractor, at the age of 31, he had a large stroke which left him with significant right-sided weakness and a severe aphasia. His wife, Mary, was thrown into a new and disturbing place: "For the first six months, it was just, it was crazy. Honestly, just like drowning." Danny's life changed completely; he was unable to work or continue with his sport and drama. He said a goal has always been: "Just talk. I just wanting talking to get better…". He added that he still finds it hard to return to previous activities: "Fringe, Shakespeare and comedy. And now I can't go to the Fringe 'cos they are laughing, and I don't know why they are laughing". By 2020, Danny and Mary have lived with aphasia for just over 20 years.

Tracey was working as a lawyer and had her stroke 14 years ago when she was just 38 years old, then married and a mother of young twins. She said of the early post stroke period: "Back then, confused, very very confused.

Depressed, a little bit suicide. My kids, three years old". Tracey has since faced many losses, including her career and her marriage, and endured years of legal battles and financial strain. Her journey has been difficult. When asked what she wanted to achieve after the first year, she said: "It's back home, it's learn driving, it's life… it's survive".

Shared goal setting

The notion of shared decision making is central to collaborative, person-centred goal setting in rehabilitation (Coulter & Collins, 2011). It rests on mutual understanding and negotiating a choice or an agreed position, and originally the models for shared decision making focused on how it occurred between individual patients and health practitioners (Charles, Gafni, & Whelan, 1997, 1999). Increasingly, there is more recognition of decisions being made collaboratively, including family, for example particularly when patients are ill or in crisis: "… the dominant view of decision making has overlooked the reality that patients, in particular, turn to others for help and support… to clinicians, who have the explicit role of offering information, advice, and support, and of course, to family members and friends" (Elwyn et al., 2014, p.159). Moreover, in clinical practice, decisions are often "contingent, tentative, and iterative" (Elwyn et al., 2014, p.160) where options are tried out and reassessed. This idea more accurately represents informal or dynamic assessments underpinning therapeutic decisions now seen within aphasia therapy (Hersh, Wood, & Armstrong, 2018). Elwyn and colleagues (2014) suggest a model of *Collaborative Deliberation* in healthcare in order to support decisions, including goal setting. This model has five related propositions: constructive engagement, recognition of alternatives, comparative learning (to compare alternative courses of action), preference construction and elicitation, and preference integration (where preferences are integrated in the plan of action). This model is flexible and recognizes that sometimes clinicians will lead, and at other times patients may take the lead.

A key problem with achieving this *shared* aspect of goal setting is that it relies on health professionals having time, communication skills and resources to inform properly and deliberate with patients and families. This, previous researchers have noted, is difficult to achieve (Brown et al., 2020; Haley et al., 2019). Patients and families often feel uninformed about the stroke, its consequences, the rehabilitation context, and aphasia itself, sometimes not even being told the word *aphasia* (Eames, Hoffmann, Worrall, & Read, 2010;

Hersh & Armstrong, 2020; Rose, Wallace, & Leow, 2019). In this situation, the chances of them being constructively engaged, able to understand alternatives or specify preferences from an informed position is very unlikely, even if they wish to do so.

Danny and Mary did not experience any sense of collaborative deliberation in the acute and sub-acute period. Mary's memory of her first impression was as follows:

> It was because he had a concussion from the stroke. That is kind of what they suggested... the doctor suggested that...

> I couldn't understand what Danny wanted, how was I going to help him? And I still didn't understand that he couldn't talk. Like it didn't hit me straight away... I just thought it was all because his head was so sore that he had this, something temporary going on. Then they said he was going to have speech therapy for his tongue to help with his tongue, so we went there and just did some mouth exercises. Only had about one or two sessions in the 30 days that we were there. And he would have physio come in and they would work on the paralysed side and then we started walking... Like I said "Danny, you are going to walk, you are going to do this, I know you can do this. We are going to do this together" and by the end of the month he started, like he just moved his leg automatically, so it started happening. And then they wanted to put him in a rehab centre which he didn't want to go to, and I didn't want because he was so young... the people that were around us were all older people that had had strokes... Danny still didn't even really understand that he had had a stroke... the whole month that we were there nobody mentioned aphasia.

Mary made sense of the situation based on those concepts with which she was already familiar – the notion of concussion, of a sore head, of a problem being temporary. She initially equated rehabilitation with older people, and therefore could not see its value for a younger person; it was unfamiliar and unexplained. Her account highlights the importance of staff explaining terminology clearly and not taking meanings for granted, particularly when families are trying to make sense of so much new information:

> I didn't understand still why couldn't he talk? I kept waiting because the doctor said "Oh, he'll probably start speaking soon" 'cos initially they said "he's not going to be able to walk..." so once he started walking, I think they got hopeful. I don't know. They didn't talk to me about anything...

What they did give me was the impression a lot of the problems he's got is because his brain is so swollen. So, I kept thinking once the swelling goes down, he's going to get back to the way he was.

And so, especially when I saw him start walking, I thought Oh OK, so everything is starting to work again. So the doctors kind of said "if you be patient I think he'll be better at this and he'll get better"… so I kind of was waiting for that and then I thought the brain must take such a long time for the swelling to go. So that is what I was waiting for because they kind of gave me the impression that when the swelling is down, he'll get a lot more movement…

So, I kept still thinking Oh, he's going to wake up one day and just start talking. Because the doctor said that that also happened to some people. He kind of would tell me "calm down about this" so I'd say "I don't understand why he can't talk". And they said "you know, we've had people like this and then once things settle down, the swelling goes down, they just start talking".

Danny's ability to recover walking gave Mary the impression that his talking would soon follow. She waited and waited for *the swelling to go down*, complying with instructions to be patient. This story shows how the brief explanations that she was given about spontaneous recovery were misunderstood because they were not given in a broader context of adequate information about stroke and aphasia. Effectively, there was no collaboration, and no early goal setting with the couple until, after six months, they happened to be seen by a speech pathologist in an outpatient community-based programme, and their experience of aphasia therapy turned a corner.

Monitored change

In the *SMARTER* framework, this aspect of goal setting is about regularly monitoring change, along the lines of the iterative process of decision making mentioned by Elwyn et al. (2014) even if it is not formally or quantitatively measured. Monitoring allows change, or lack of change, to be discussed and noted to help inform what to do next. While clear evidence of change on outcome measures is crucial to check treatment effectiveness and direction, meaningful changes can also be picked up and documented through client and family self-evaluation. This feature of the model highlights the importance of keeping track in various ways so that intervention is well targeted, agreed and re-directed as appropriate.

Tracey's account of her therapy over a number of years revealed how this process of monitoring looked for her in a real-world context. She described wanting ongoing speech therapy because she felt, without it, her language skills deteriorated. Private therapy was too expensive, so she attended a university clinic and was grateful to receive therapy there from students working under supervision.

> DH: When you go and see the students for speech therapy, does anybody there say what would you like to work on?
>
> T: Yes.
>
> DH: So, tell me about that.
>
> T: Well, goals, you know. And, well, she says, you know… Tracey goals and session and then… construct a sentence and I have a problem with the verbs and prepositions. And pronouns and sometimes "there's a woman…"
>
> DH: Oh, with the clause…
>
> T: Yeah… sometimes it's erm… pictures.
>
> DH: Sequences. So, putting those together into longer sequences?
>
> T: Yes.
>
> DH: OK. Alright. I mean, do you… how do you feel about the goals that they're working towards?
>
> T: Erm… goals er… not really, but speech therapy goals… because I am happy it's, you know, I am happy erm… it's like construct a sentence.
>
> DH: Do you have that feeling like "at least I'm getting some therapy"?
>
> T: Yeah. Exactly. Because, because it's… I know erm aphasia, it's back to six months or one year it's no therapy.
>
> DH: So at least you've got something now from the university?
>
> T: Because so expensive, private. Speech therapy. So expensive.
>
> DH: Do you have other goals to work towards or other ideas about what you would like to do in therapy or are they the same as what they want to do?
>
> T: It's different styles… three students to one and then change, different

students, personality, you know?

DH: So, you only have them for short amounts of time.

T: Six weeks or seven weeks. One hour a week.

DH: Yeah, and then when new students start after the term, do you go through that goal setting discussion again?

T: Oh, yeah. Yeah.

DH: And does it change what you then do with them?

T: No.

DH: You still end up doing the same therapy?

T: Yeah.

DH So each group of students that you've seen, have they all been working on sentences?

T: Two years.

DH: For two years. Sentence construction and the grammar, grammatical sentence building.

T: Yeah.

DH: How do you feel about that?

T: Erm… well, with me happy construct a sentence.

DH: Yes, it is a good thing for you to work on.

T: Yes. Or I quit speech therapy two years or three years and I've lost.

DH: So, you felt your language went backwards when you weren't having it?

T: Yep…

DH: Do you have thoughts about what you would like to achieve with your language in a year's time?

T: No because it's different students.

DH: There isn't that continuity?

T: No. If I have one speech therapy, yes, one goal, three goals.

This excerpt of our discussion demonstrates the nuanced nature of these issues. Tracey was involved in goal setting discussions with the students, but she felt they always seemed to yield the same impairment-focused approach to her agrammatic expressive output. While Tracey believed she was making progress, that she needed to keep going, and was positive about working with students, the monitoring of change and planning for the longer term seemed to have gone awry because of the term-by-term nature of the therapy, always a new start for each group of students, but not for her.

Accessibility

This feature of *SMARTER* is about ensuring the process of setting goals is accessible or *aphasia friendly*. This includes being aware that the concept of a goal means different things to different people (Hersh et al., 2012b). Accessibility applies to the way goals are discussed, validating understanding, presenting information and choices with visual supports, using decision-aids, and documenting in such a way as to allow further deliberation as well as for the formal record. Considering the process may involve negotiating long-term goals being split into short-term goals, this may be a complex set of ideas to convey. Danny and Mary remember therapy stopped feeling formulaic and that goal setting became both meaningful and accessible at six months post stroke once they started working with their new community therapist, Amy (pseudonym). Mary said:

> I found the difference… I just found that a few therapists we had at the beginning did everything almost like a textbook: *has a stroke, has aphasia so do flashcards, do this…* They both did exactly the same thing without (involving) either one of us. But when we got to Amy the reason it felt different was because it didn't feel like it was a classroom or a therapy session and that was because she first had to understand who Danny was.

For Tracey, accessibility has been a fundamental issue in trying to receive therapy at all. She reported being frustrated for a while by the Australian National Disability Insurance Scheme (NDIS), a potential avenue to financial access for a wider range of therapy services. She struggled to navigate the complex documentation and the processes as someone with aphasia living alone. Tracey said this process was "huge, very very stress". She was initially refused funding, including having her appeal declined: "I think it's NDIS, it's squeezing financial". More recently, Tracey has been successful in securing funding from the NDIS, has now finished therapy at the university clinic and has started private speech therapy. Tracey's story highlights the need to be able to access services in the first place, sometimes a difficult task. Now with funding, she has her 'one speech therapy' and is able to negotiate a tailored plan for the longer term.

Relevance

Therapy goals need to be relevant to patients and families. Clearly, there is little point investing time in an intervention that is not useful or applicable. Negotiating relevant goals depends on moving beyond therapy developed from seeing where the deficits show up in an assessment, but relies instead on having some common ground, shared understandings, and knowledge about the current circumstances and concerns of the patient and family. Tracey mentioned examples where her speech pathologists focused directly on important areas relevant to her, particularly early on, with her ability to talk to her children and to manage as they started school. However, at other times she has had to find alternative support, for example going to a friend to get help with letters and documents as she went through the Family Court, or later negotiating the NDIS.

Mary noted how irrelevant goals were essentially demotivating:

He (Danny) was just very mellow and he didn't apply himself because all we were doing was flashcards. I think he said one day he felt like he was starting kindergarten again. He couldn't understand and I didn't understand why we were using flashcards. I still don't to this day to be honest. I mean I understand why visuals were good, but I didn't understand why looking at a coat and a goat was important.

On the other hand, with Amy, the work changed, and their level of engagement changed:

She just tapped into him so quick. She got him to respond, for the first time since his stroke, he was animated, and I was like "he is understanding!" So that is why I went every day and… I would do things that she did at home, and I would tell everybody at home: If you ask him something keep it simple and he might only pick up two or three things so emphasise things you want and this and that. But then Amy started doing things like finding out his interests. And when she found out he was a football fanatic, which I know she hated, she started learning about football. So, she would start sessions with "oh, geez Dan, bad week for the footy team this week!" So, it would start automatically and from there she would start going into therapy. And he kind of didn't really notice the difference, do you know what I mean? And then they would talk about things. That's when he started responding because she would bring in his interests, about the theatre especially, and the football and that would make the speech therapy session. And so that level of frustration started going away.

Transparent

This feature of the framework is about whether there are clear links between people's life goals (Nair, 2003), long-term rehabilitation goals, small goals/steps, and actual therapy tasks and activities. These links may need to be highlighted explicitly because unless there is a rationale for effort, motivation wanes. Tracey was keen to continue her therapy with the university, but the transparency of links between her speech therapy and her personal goals was a little cloudy because of the continuous renegotiation of similar goals set with students. She noted a few of her life goals: "It's planning… erm… 65, it's my backyard, granny flat or subdivide… it's me… and now financial. I have determine, you know".

Mary noted, early on, that she did not really understand the importance placed on goal setting in relation to choices in therapy, or even in planning for services. Later, she was concerned that the implications of goal setting were not made transparent, for example describing feeling fearful that if Danny did not meet a goal, that he might be judged negatively and risk losing funding and opportunities for further therapy. Mary's point highlights why collaboration is so important: not only does the process of goal setting have links to short- and long-term goals and to therapy choices and direction, but it also has the potential to influence the length, intensity and even availability of a service. Such important decisions should rest on a clear and transparent process.

Evolving

People's goals change over time, particularly long stretches of time as for Danny, Mary and Tracey. Quite separately from the short-term cycles of goal setting Tracey experienced, her life goals appear to be shifting over time. Tracey has joined the committee of a State support and advocacy organization for people with aphasia. Mary became more assertive about demanding services after realising the benefits of having the right therapist:

> We fought so long to keep Amy. 'Cos they only gave us like six-month sessions, and I said "no, he is responding like you wouldn't believe" so I fought everybody on it and for two years we managed to do like four sessions six months each time. After that they wouldn't let us do any more rehab even though they saw the difference themselves... So, then we started doing it privately because I said there is no way I am letting Amy go now that she knows how to tap into everything, and I was seeing all the results. But they didn't believe that he could do any better. And he did. And I had to explain that to one of the women that rejected... she works in the Department of Disability... And I said "oh, you're not going to like me very much 'cos I reckon you got a lot of my phone calls and letters... you guys cut off these people without even really seeing them... I am sorry but you are going to listen because there are so many people, they are nonverbal, and they can't fight for themselves. How dare you cut them off from the only people that can help them?"

This example shows that goals may be about benefiting the community. People with aphasia and families will develop ideas about what they want to achieve in response to new information, new experiences and changing demands. Danny and Mary learned of the importance of understanding aphasia, and of raising awareness of aphasia. They responded to their situation by giving their time and effort to assist others in a similar situation through their local aphasia support organization, organizing and disseminating the newsletter to the membership.

The journeys described here reflect the findings of recent research. Wray and Clarke (2017) carried out a systematic review of the longer-term needs of people with communication difficulties after stroke living in the community. Their synthesis of 32 qualitative studies showed that challenges existed for many years after the stroke, particularly impacting on social networks and participation. Four themes relating to longer-term need were: managing communication outside of the home; creating a meaningful role; sustaining the support network; and feeling empowered to move forward. These authors suggested that interventions for self-management are important. Their work raises questions about whether aphasia clinicians should consider advocacy and self-management goals more actively in the longer term, a point also made by Nichol et al. (2019). Manning and colleagues (2019) also carried out a systematic review and qualitative evidence synthesis of what influences recovery and living successfully with aphasia. They reported five themes: family and friends of people with aphasia also require support; there is a need to contribute to society and be part of it; enabling environments and opportunities are important; ongoing services should be flexible and relevant; and people with aphasia and their families should be empowered to navigate the health system through information and collaborative interactions with healthcare professionals. These themes resonate strongly with the experiences reported for Tracey, Danny and Mary. They all contribute positively within their own communities and have called for better, more flexible systems of support, whether financial or legal, for people with chronic aphasia.

Relationship centred

Finally, the SMARTER framework recognizes the centrality of relationships in goal setting, and how sensitivity, respect and a deep knowledge of the needs of a patient and family can assist the renegotiation of goals over time (Bright, Kayes, Cummins, Worrall, & McPherson, 2017; Fourie, 2009, Worrall et al., 2011). Danny and Mary's relationship with Amy opened doors to them: to understanding the aphasia; to relevant, meaningful therapy; to the opportunity to contribute to therapy direction; to engage and see progress. In their work on the therapeutic alliance, Lawton, Haddock, Conroy, Serrant & Sage (2018) note its importance for goal agreement, collaborative engagement required for therapeutic tasks, and an interpersonal bond. A therapeutic alliance contributes to self-efficacy, treatment outcome, adherence, and satisfaction. Lawton et al. (2018) discussed *readiness*, seeing a point to the alliance and to therapy. This was more likely if people understood their situation and their diagnosis, and if there was collaborative engagement which encompassed participants' desire to assume ownership over their therapy.

Conclusion

This chapter has brought together research and real-world experiences to explore goal setting in aphasia therapy. Using the *SMARTER* goal setting framework (Hersh et al., 2012a), we have illustrated that goal setting for aphasia therapy, whether in acute, sub-acute or chronic phases of aphasia recovery, demands information sharing, clear discussions about change, or lack of it, excellent accessible communication, clarity, transparency, and a respectful relationship. The overview of research in the introduction suggested clinicians were often unable to secure sufficient time to achieve collaborative goal setting and that non-speech pathologists might not have the confidence to manage the supported communication strategies involved. However, time and good communication are an investment in goal setting. A collaborative process underpins a potentially more successful therapeutic journey and is worth the extra preparation in the longer term. Mary's contribution to this chapter also highlights the need to include and support family members because their ability to contribute effectively to goal setting and therapy is enhanced when they understand and can be part of collaborative deliberation (Howe et al., 2012). Our perspectives have been presented as narratives to help sensitize readers to the impact of goal setting and subsequent therapy direction, not only in early rehabilitation but well into the chronic phase. We suggest that, for people whose lives are changed dramatically with the onset of aphasia, how goal setting is done reflects the quality of the subsequent therapy. It needs to be an informative and useful process, built from a strong relationship, helping to link therapy tasks with short- and long-term planning, sufficiently flexible to change with time, and a process that supports people with aphasia and their families to move on successfully.

Acknowledgements

We would like to thank Jan Rolan for her helpful and insightful comments on this chapter.

References

Alanko, T., Karhula, M., Kröger, T., Piirainen, A., & Nikander, R. (2019). Rehabilitees perspective on goal setting in rehabilitation – a phenomenological approach. *Disability and Rehabilitation, 41*(19), 2280-2288. doi:10.1080/09638288.2018.1463398

Barnard, R.A., Cruice, M., & Playford, E.D. (2010). Strategies used in the pursuit of achievability during goal setting in rehabilitation. *Qualitative Health Research, 20*(2), 239-250. doi:10.1177/1049732309358327.

Berg, K., Rise, M.B., Balandin, S., Armstrong, E., Askim, T. (2016). Speech pathologists' experience of involving people with stroke-induced aphasia in clinical decision making during rehabilitation. *Disability and Rehabilitation, 38*(9), 870-878. doi:10.3109/0963 8288.2015.1066453

Berg, K., Askim, T., Balandin, S., Armstrong, E., Rise, M.B. (2017). Experiences of participation in goal setting for people with stroke-induced aphasia in Norway. A qualitative study. *Disability and Rehabilitation, 39*(11), 1122-1130. doi:10.1080/0963 8288.2016.1185167

Bright, F.A.S., Kayes, N.M., Cummins, C., Worrall, L.M. & McPherson, K.M. (2017). Co-constructing engagement in stroke rehabilitation: A qualitative study exploring how practitioner engagement can influence patient engagement. *Clinical Rehabilitation, 31*(10), 1396-1405. doi:10.1177/0269215517694678

Brown, S.E., Brady, M.C., Worrall, L., & Scobbie, L. (2021). A narrative review of communication accessibility for people with aphasia and implications for multi-disciplinary goal setting after stroke. *Aphasiology, 35*(1), 1-32. doi:10.1080/02687038.2020.1759269

Brown, M., Levack, W., McPherson, K.M., Dean, S.G., Reed, K., Weatherall, M., & Taylor, W.J. (2014). Survival, momentum, and things that make me "me": Patients' perceptions of goal setting after stroke. *Disability and Rehabilitation, 36*(12), 1020-1026. doi:10.31 09/09638288.2013.825653

Charles, C., Gafni A., & Whelan, T. (1997). Shared decision-making in the medical encounter: What does it mean? (or it takes at least two to tango). *Social Science and Medicine, 44*(5), 681–692. doi:10.1016/s0277-9536(96)00221-3

Charles, C., Gafni A., &Whelan, T. (1999). Decision-making in the physician–patient encounter: Revisiting the shared treatment decision-making model. *Social Science and Medicine, 49*(5), 651–661. doi:10.1016/s0277-9536(99)00145-8

Coulter, A. & Collins, A. (2011). *Making Shared Decision-Making a Reality: No Decision About Me Without Me.* London, UK: The King's Fund.

Eames, S., Hoffmann, T., Worrall, L., & Read, S. (2010). Stroke patients' and carers' perception of barriers to accessing stroke information. *Topics in Stroke Rehabilitation, 17*, 69-78. doi:10.1310/tsr1702-69

Elston, A., Barnden, R., Hersh, D., Godecke, E., Cadilhac, D., Lannin, N., Kneebone, I., & Andrew, N. (2021). Developing person-centred goal setting resources with and for people with aphasia: A multi-phase qualitative study. *Aphasiology.* https://doi.org/10.1080/02687038.2021.1907294

Elwyn, G., Lloyd, A., May, C., van der Weijden, T., Stiggelbout, A., Edwards, A., Frosch, D.L., Rapley, T., Barr, P., Walsh, T., Grande, S.W., Montori, V., & Epstein, R. (2014). Collaborative deliberation: A model for patient care. *Patient Education and Counseling, 97*(2), 158-164. doi:10.1016/j.pec.2014.07.027

Fourie, R.J. (2009). Qualitative study of the therapeutic relationship in speech and language therapy: Perspectives of adults with acquired communication and swallowing disorders. *International Journal of Language and Communication Disorders, 44*(6), 979-999. doi: 10.1080/13682820802535285.

Franklin, M., Lewis, S., Willis, K., Rogers, A., Venville, A., & Smith, L. (2019). Controlled, constrained, or flexible? How self-management goals are shaped by patient-provider interactions. *Qualitative Health Research, 29*(4), 557-567. doi:10.1177/1049732318774324

Hayley, K.L., Cunningham, K.T., Barry, J., & de Riesthal, M. (2019). Collaborative goals for communicative life participation in aphasia: The FOURC Model. *American Journal of Speech-Language Pathology, 28*(1), 1-13. https://doi.org/10.1044/2018_AJSLP-18-0163

Hersh, D. & Armstrong, E. (2020). Information, communication, advocacy, and complaint: How the spouse of a man with aphasia managed his discharge from hospital. *Aphasiology.* https://doi.org/10.1080/02687038.2020.1765304

Hersh, D., Worrall, L., Howe, T., Sherratt, S., & Davidson, B. (2012a). SMARTER goal setting in aphasia rehabilitation. *Aphasiology, 26*(2), 220-233. http://dx.doi.org/10.10 80/02687038.2011.640392

Hersh, D., Sherratt, S., Howe, T., Worrall, L., Davidson, B., & Ferguson, A. (2012b). An analysis of the "goal" in aphasia rehabilitation. *Aphasiology, 26*(8), 971-984. http://dx.doi. org/10.1080/02687038.2012.684339

Hersh, D., Wood, P., & Armstrong, E. (2018). Informal aphasia assessment, interaction and the development of the therapeutic relationship in the early period after stroke. *Aphasiology, 32*(8), 876-901. https://doi.org/10.1080/02687038.2017.1381878

Howe, T., Davidson, B., Worrall, L., Hersh, D., Ferguson, A., Sherratt, S. & Gilbert, J. (2012). 'You needed to rehab… families as well': Family members' own goals for aphasia rehabilitation. *International Journal of Language and Communication Disorders, 47*(5), 511-521. doi:10.1111/j.1460-6984.2012.00159.x

Lawton, M., Haddock, G., Conroy, P., Serrant, L., & Sage, K. (2018). People with aphasia's perception of the therapeutic alliance in aphasia rehabilitation post stroke: A thematic analysis. *Aphasiology, 32*(12), 1397-1417. doi:10.1080/02687038.2018.1441365

Leach, E., Cornwell, P., Fleming, J., & Haines, T. (2010). Patient centered goal-setting in a subacute rehabilitation setting. *Disability and Rehabilitation, 32*(2), 159-172. doi:10.3109/09638280903036605

Levack, W.M. & Siegert, J. (2015). Challenges in theory, practice and evidence. In: R.J. Siegert & W. Levack. (Eds), *Rehabilitation Goal Setting: Theory, Practice and Evidence* (pp.3-19). London, UK: Taylor & Francis.

Levack, W.M., Dean, S.G., McPherson, K., & Siegert, J. (2015). Evidence-based goal setting: Cultivating the science of rehabilitation. In: R.J. Siegert & W. Levack (Eds), *Rehabilitation Goal Setting: Theory, Practice and Evidence* (pp.21-44). London, UK: Taylor & Francis.

Levack, W.M., Dean, S.G., Siegert, R.J., & McPherson, K.M. (2011). Navigating patient-centered goal setting in inpatient stroke rehabilitation: How clinicians control the process to meet perceived professional responsibilities. *Patient Education & Counseling, 85*(2), 206-213. doi:10.1016/j.pec.2011.01.011

Levack, W., Weatherall, M., Hay-Smith, E., Dean, S.G., McPherson, K., & Siegert, R.J. (2015). Goal setting and strategies to enhance goal pursuit for adults with acquired disability participating in rehabilitation. *Cochrane Database of Systematic Reviews, 7*, CD009727. https://doi.org/10.1002/14651858.CD009727.pub2

Manning, M., MacFarlane, A., Hickey, A., & Franklin, S. (2019.) Perspectives of people with aphasia post-stroke towards personal recovery and living successfully: A systematic review and thematic synthesis. *PLoS ONE, 14*(3), e0214200. https://doi.org/10.1371/ journal.pone.0214200

Nair, K.P. . (2003). Life goals: The concept and its relevance to rehabilitation. *Clinical Rehabilitation, 17*(2), 192–202. https://doi.org/10.1191/0269215503cr599oa

National Health and Medical Research Council. (2019). Authorship: A guide supporting the Australian Code for the Responsible Conduct of Research: R41C. National Health and Medical Research Council, Australian Research Council and Universities Australia. Commonwealth of Australia, Canberra. ISBN Online: 978-1-86496-034-1

Nichol, L., Hill, A.J., Wallace, S.J., Pitt, R., Baker, C., & Rodriguez, A.D. (2019). Self-management of aphasia: A scoping review. *Aphasiology, 33*(8), 903–942. doi:10.1080/02687038.2019.1575065

Parry, R.H. (2004). Communication during goal-setting in physiotherapy treatment sessions. *Clinical Rehabilitation, 18*(6), 668–682. doi:10.1191/0269215504cr745oa

Rohde, A., Townley-O'Neill, K., Trendall, K., Worrall, L., & Cornwell, P. (2012). A comparison of client and therapist goals for people with aphasia: A qualitative exploratory study. *Aphasiology, 26*(10), 1298–1315. doi:10.1080/02687038.2012.706799

Rose, T., Wallace, S., & Leow, S. (2019). Family members' experiences and preferences for receiving aphasia information during early phases in the continuum of care. *International Journal of Speech-Language Pathology, 21*, 470–482. doi:10.1080/17549507.2019.1651396

Rosewilliam, S., Roskell, C.A., & Pandyan, A.D. (2011). A systematic review and synthesis of the quantitative and qualitative evidence behind patient-centred goal setting in stroke rehabilitation. *Clinical Rehabilitation, 25*(6), 501–514. doi:10.1177/0269215510394467

Schut, H.A. & Stam, H.J. (1994). Goals in rehabilitation teamwork. *Disability and Rehabilitation, 16*(4), 223–226. doi:10.3109/09638289409166616.

Scobbie, L., Thomson, K., Pollock, A., & Evans, J. (2020). Goal adjustment by people living with long-term conditions: A scoping review of literature published from January 2007 to June 2018. *Neuropsychological Rehabilitation.* doi:10.1080/09602011.2020.1774397

Sherratt, S., Worrall, L., Pearson, C., Howe, T., Hersh, D., & Davidson, B. (2011). "Well it has to be language-related": Speech-language pathologists' goals for people with aphasia and their families. *International Journal of Speech-Language Pathology, 13*(4), 317–328. doi:10.3109/17549507.2011.584632

Sugavanam, T., Mead, G., Bulley, C., Donaghy, M., & van Wijck, F. (2013). The effects and experiences of goal setting in stroke rehabilitation - a systematic review. *Disability and Rehabilitation, 35*(3), 177–190. doi:10.3109/09638288.2012.690501

Worrall, L., Davidson, B., Hersh, D., Ferguson, A., Howe, T., & Sherratt, S. (2010). The evidence for relationship-centred practice in aphasia rehabilitation. *Journal of Interactional Research in Communication Disorders, 1*(2), 277-300. https://doi.org/10.1558/jircd.v1i2.277

Worrall, L., Sherratt, S., Rogers, P., Howe, T., Hersh, D., & Ferguson, A. (2011). What people with aphasia want: Their goals according to the ICF. *Aphasiology, 25*(3), 309–322. https://doi.org/10.1080/02687038.2010.508530

Wray, F. & Clarke, D. (2017). Longer-term needs of stroke survivors with communication difficulties living in the community: a systematic review and thematic synthesis of qualitative studies. *BMJ Open, 7*, e017944. doi:10.1136/ bmjopen-2017-017944

2 Reframing aphasia assessment: A principled and practical approach

Jen Thomson

> Assessment is not an end in itself but must be considered in relation to its potential value to the patient. (Spreen & Risser, 2003, p.223)

Introduction

My interest in assessment practice began over a decade ago, after one particular clinical experience in the early days of my work as a Speech & Language Therapist (SLT). I started to support a retired businessman who had been living with severe aphasia for several years at home with his wife. His case had been passed on to me after initial assessment sessions with a colleague. When reading through his notes, I was struck that formal assessment seemed to be the sole focus of these sessions and, contrary to my relatively recent university training, the results seemed somewhat limited in their clinical value (beyond outlining his deficits). I felt left with more questions than answers. Was formal 'testing' the best option? Did the assessment really capture his communication strengths? How did it capture the impact of aphasia upon his everyday life? Was the assessment related to his goals and did it inform how to support them? Was the purpose of the assessment clear? How did it reflect the role and value of Speech & Language Therapy?

Answers to traditional questions about assessment are well established. Why do SLTs assess? To gather information on linguistic and communicative strengths and weaknesses, to enable diagnosis and severity of the aphasia, to identify relationships to theoretical frameworks and potential intervention options, as well as use as outcome measurement. When do we assess? At the beginning of an intervention period, typically before 'therapy'. How do we assess? By using a wide range of informal and formal assessment approaches, methods, and tools with suitability determined by the SLT.

Whilst these answers hold true, for me, they don't fully address the questions arising from that early clinical experience – questions about assessment ethos, value, and what can be described generally as 'the black box' of assessment practice, i.e., 'the doing'. Over the last ten years, I have been motivated to try and seek more clinically satisfying answers. In doing so, a particular approach to aphasia assessment has emerged within my own practice. In brief, the approach centres around assessment as a therapeutic activity; informal, discourse-based assessment being the primary focus of the assessment encounter, and formal, test-based assessment being aligned to a person's goals. This chapter is an opportunity to share how this approach is framed, structured and is guided by the evidence base. It creates space for reflection for SLTs with an already similar assessment practice, and acts as a way-marker for SLTs drawn to move towards using such an assessment approach. Part I provides an overview of the approach and its informing principles, with Part II focusing on more practical guidance.

Part I: Assessment approach

The approach has two phases:

- Establishing Assessment
- Goal-focused Assessment.

Establishing Assessment is the primary assessment phase. It refers to the process by which the SLT broadly establishes a person with aphasia's communicative performance and proficiency from the first moments of clinical interaction, 'optimising the initial contact' (as stated by the Australian Aphasia Rehabilitation Pathway (CCREIAR, 2014)). It uses semi-structured interviewing and/or conversation as the main assessment method, with the SLT creating more naturalistic opportunities to elicit certain communication behaviours and opportunities for information exchange. Elicitation via intentional and abstracted 'testing' – either formal or informal – is minimized at this early stage. The aim is still to identify the presence/absence of aphasia, communicative strengths and difficulties, barriers and facilitators to communication, the impact of the communication disorder upon 'real life', as well as the person's communication goals. The method requires the SLT to be confident in: (a) clinical knowledge of the relevant communication skills and information that requires exploration during the semi-structured interview/conversation; and (b) clinical skill in *how* to best explore the relevant aspects within the semi-structured interview/conversation, in a systematic, yet naturalistic manner. The process may take several sessions, or be readily achieved with a single session, dependent on the individual.

Goal-focused Assessment is the secondary assessment phase. It refers to a more detailed and in-depth evaluation of communicative ability relating only to a specific need or goal, as identified by the person with aphasia. This phase therefore happens *after* goal setting conversations, and only if the necessary information has not been adequately gained during Establishing Assessment. Informal and formal methods (including 'testing') are appropriate here – the SLT needs to determine which approach and tools are most suitable on a case-by-case basis. Goal-focused Assessment can be brief, occur within the same session as Establishing Assessment or can take several sessions to fully explore performance and inform intervention options relating to a goal, in collaboration with the person with aphasia.

Establishing Assessment and Goal-focused Assessment are both highly principled. The phases are informed by a set of principles that have emerged from the aphasia literature over recent years, making clear a contemporary view on the purpose of assessment and how assessment sits in the wider context of aphasia management. These principles are reflected in several clinical guidance documents, e.g., Australian Aphasia Rehabilitation Pathway Supplementary Best Practice Statements (CCREIAR, 2014) and The Top Ten: Best Practice Recommendations for Aphasia (Simmons-Mackie et al., 2017). These principles also emerged from our scoping review of the informal aphasia assessment literature (Thomson, Gee, Sage, & Walker, 2018). Fundamental guiding principles include:

1. Assessment is a therapeutic intervention in its own right.

2. Assessment should reflect performance of real-world communication.

3. Assessment should include the impact of aphasia on everyday life.

4. Assessment should relate to the needs and goals of the person with aphasia.

Assessment also needs to be efficient, effective and demonstrate the specialist value and role of the SLT. In the current context of healthcare provision 'every contact has to count'. SLTs often report time pressures and competing clinical demands, e.g., swallowing versus communication intervention (Foster, Worrall, Rose, & O'Halloran, 2016). Assessment needs to be a highly informative process for all involved – the SLT, the person with aphasia, their family/carers and the wider care team. SLTs have to ensure that the service they are offering benefits the person with aphasia by maximizing the wealth of specialist skill and knowledge held only by the SLT. The guiding principles, outlined in more detail below, support these aims.

1. Assessment is a therapeutic intervention in its own right

Assessment can be no longer seen as separate to therapy; it is a therapeutic intervention in itself. Several factors make assessment a therapeutic process – articulated particularly by Hersh and colleagues (2012, 2013, 2017). These include:

- *Active engagement*: The person with aphasia (and often their family or carer) is actively engaged in the process (Hersh, Worrall, O'Halloran, Brown, Grohn, & Rodriguez, 2013). Bright, Kayes, Worrall & McPherson (2015) propose engagement to be a co-constructed process, which enables the individual to become an active, committed and invested collaborator in healthcare through the gradual connection between the individual, the clinician and/or a therapeutic programme.

- *Information sharing*: The SLT shares information during the encounter that may enable the person with aphasia to better understand their condition and situation, e.g., their medical condition, communication diagnosis, the rehabilitation process, the impact of the disorder (Hersh et al., 2013).

- *Identifying needs, wants and goals*: The SLT readily explores and supports the person with aphasia in identifying their needs, wants and goals during the process, supported by the assessment methodology selected. For example, many of the inherent qualities of informal assessment allow greater opportunity for the person with aphasia to collaborate with the SLT (Hersh, Worrall, Howe, Sherratt & Davison, 2012; see also Chapter 1 in this book).

- *Communicative success* and *experimenting with communication support*: The SLT experiments *dynamically* with factors that may influence performance during the assessment (e.g., communication strategies, task modification, context factors and environmental supports (Coelho, Ylvisaker & Turkstra, 2005)). This is known as process-based assessment and is often referred to as 'dynamic assessment'. The person with aphasia is less constrained or limited to a given (language) task or activity based on a binary 'correct' or 'incorrect' response.

- *Supporting the development of a therapeutic relationship*: In their recent metasynthesis exploring therapeutic relationships for those with communication impairments after stroke, Bright and Reeves (2020) reinforce the need for clinicians to see the development of the therapeutic relationship as an integral part of the rehabilitation process. The authors highlight how the interaction between the client and clinician is critical in building this relationship, and identify core characteristics of communication that foster therapeutic relationships, including reflecting the 'human' needs of the individual (Pound & Jensen, 2018). The impact of an assessment encounter and its processes upon the development of the therapeutic relationship is worth consideration; minimizing interactions that can foster 'therapeutic disconnection' (Bright & Reeves, 2020) and capitalizing on opportunities to foster the therapeutic relationships, e.g., recognizing personhood, sharing expectations, encouraging role ownership and therapeutic responsiveness (Lawton, Sage, Conroy, & Serrant, 2018a; Lawton, Haddock, Conroy, Serrant, & Sage, 2018b). This endeavour can influence the assessment method selected, with Hersh, Wood and Armstrong (2017) concluding that the choices made to assess informally are "as much about balancing clinician-centred and client-centred interactions, and the management or facilitation of relationships, as about use of non-standardised tools and flexible tasks" (Hersh et al., 2017, p.24). The authors refer to the wider rehabilitation literature to highlight how a move to a more conversational assessment methodology encourages a 'shift in the usual power structure' of clinical interactions' (Togher, 2003, p. 7).

> ### Process-based assessment: The importance of learning
>
> The case for process-based assessment has its origins in the paediatric literature – stemming from dissatisfaction with standardized testing processes. For example, a static measure can usefully measure a child's vocabulary but not their ability to learn words.
>
> A process-based assessment approach is interested in exploring the learning process during assessment. Several techniques can be used, e.g., graduated prompting or a test-teach-test paradigm. This learning information is then used to inform wider management, e.g., therapy design, treatment decisions and potential responsiveness to therapy (Kelley & Goldstein, 2019).
>
> In 'Assess for Success', Hersh et al. (2013) discuss the importance of learning theory more broadly in assessment. They suggest adults want to know why they are learning something before undertaking it and expect that learning to be useful and relevant to their lives. Providing a score is therefore not enough for assessment outcome. The process needs to inform the person with aphasia about what the information gained will contribute that is relevant to them and how the information will be used.

2. Assessment reflecting performance of real-world communication

Ecologically valid assessments demonstrate how a communication problem is naturally displayed in the 'here and now' of everyday communication. This is compared to performance on artificial assessments (e.g., tests) that are abstracted away from real-world communication activities. People with aphasia display their aphasia differently in naturalistic contexts compared to those that are more artificial, and certain communicative performances are known to be demonstrated only within naturalistic communicative contexts, such as conversation (Armstrong & Mortensen, 2006; Beeke, Wilkinson, & Maxim, 2003; Herbert, Hickin, Howard, Osborne, & Best, 2008; Jaecks, Hielscher-Fastabend, & Stenneken, 2012). Conversational discourse is then an ecologically valid assessment method to be sampled in clinical contexts, as it is the most frequent and natural communication activity that best reflects real-life communication (more than language testing) (Armstrong, 2000; Hesketh, Long, Patchick, Lee, & Bowen, 2008; Ramsberger & Rende, 2002).

Yet clinical discourse-based assessment is not without its challenges. Performance data from everyday conversations between the SLT and person with aphasia are not automatically transferable to the individual's conversations in their everyday lives, due to factors such as the SLT's experience of aphasia and skill in supported conversation (Myrberg, Hyden, & Samuelsson, 2017). Fully understanding communication in the real world – in terms of the numerous aspects that are at play in naturalistic communication – also poses a significant challenge for SLTs. The very aspects which influence everyday communicative ability are not yet fully understood, but are being explored, e.g., defining 'situated' language use (Doedens & Meteyard, 2018) and capturing face-to-face (termed 'co-present') communication (Barnes & Bloch, 2019). Furthermore, there can be lack of clinical procedural rigour in discourse assessment. Armstrong, Brady, Mackenzie and Norrie (2007) explored transcription-less methods of discourse analysis and raise lack of accuracy with these methods; however, they do suggest accuracy can be achieved with experience and training in analysis methods. Bryant, Ferguson and Spencer (2016) found subjective, judgement-based analysis to be the most frequent discourse analysis method used by clinicians (compared to detailed linguistic analysis). The authors do comment on continued use of these methods given SLTs' value in using them, and recognize the demands of the clinical setting in contributing to adaptations in linguistic discourse analysis.

> **NB:** It is worth stating that the informal, discourse-based approach used in Establishing Assessment (described in more detailed later in the chapter), does use a transcription-less approach and judgement-based analysis but if discourse is identified as a goal by the person with aphasia then a more formal and detailed approach to discourse sampling, transcription and analysis is recommended in order to capture change at the level of discourse.

3. Assessment including of the impact of aphasia upon everyday life

The initial assessment of a person with aphasia strongly influences the SLT's subsequent choice of therapy objectives, intervention approaches and what aspects are measured (Kagan & Simmons-Mackie, 2007). Assessment should then reflect the ultimate aim of SLT intervention: facilitation in life participation by people with aphasia. Kagan and Simmons-Mackie (2007) argue that choice of assessment method and intervention offered by SLTs should focus on meaningful 'end' goals relating to life participation by "beginning at the end" – a value that defines a highly effective aphasia SLT, as described by people with aphasia and their families (Worrall, 2019). The impact of aphasia upon a person's everyday life – their activity, participation and wellbeing – then needs to be established along with the nature and severity of their language problem, e.g., their impairment (Davidson & Worrall, 2000). Establishing a person with aphasia's abilities and behaviours across *all* aspects of the World Health Organisation's International Classification of Functioning, Disability and Health (ICF) (WHO, 2001) is argued to be "imperative for meaningful outcomes in aphasia" (Armstrong, Bryant, Ferguson, & Simmons-Mackie, 2016, p.271).

It should be noted that the ICF is not without constructive challenge as a supportive framework for assessment practice. Barnes and Bloch (2019), in their work exploring why measuring co-present (face-to-face) communication is so problematic, suggest the ICF still promotes an individual locus for communication and that mapping communication phenomena with the activity component has proven troublesome. The authors argue that SLTs must be equipped with relevant conceptual frameworks that allow for real-time co-present communication measurement. They introduce parts of a conceptual framework to help elaborate the use of the ICF for this purpose (see Barnes & Bloch (2019) for a comprehensive explanation).

4. Assessment relating to the needs and goals of the person with aphasia

SLTs can meet the challenge set by Kagan and Simmons-Mackie (2007) – of beginning with the end in mind – by viewing assessment as *the process which identifies and informs how best to address the person with aphasia's current needs and goals* (Hinckley, 2017). This shift in clinical thinking leads to a radically different approach for the assessment process. In this approach, the person with aphasia and their family are asked about rehabilitation priorities, goals, valued activities and life participation *prior* to any (formal) assessment. These aspects then drive the assessment process – any in/formal assessments are only used if they directly relate to and inform the skill and strategy requirements for their identified priorities, goals, valued activities. This position goes on to be reflected in the therapy approach, with therapy selection also mapping clearly onto the priorities and values of the person with aphasia and their family (Hinckley, 2017).

This shift undoubtedly leads to the capturing of different information, with varying amounts of detail, for certain aspects of a person's language and communication than they may be used to. It also challenges for whose benefit assessment information is being sought. For example, exploring reading and writing ability in depth can be seen as questionable, for several reasons, if the person with aphasia states they have no goals linked to reading and writing. This view promotes the person with aphasia working in collaboration with the SLT, identifying what is of value at a given time point. It can lead to concern from the SLT that a person with aphasia may not fully realize the potential impact upon activity and participation if certain abilities are not fully explored during assessment, with resultant consequence (e.g., access to services). Whilst this is true, the challenge is to assess the degree of information that is required, and the manner in which it is obtained, to inform the person with aphasia and their family about any potential impact of aphasia upon their everyday life. This is also the case for information to share with the wider care team and to guide potential next steps (e.g., the selection of suitable therapies to meet a specific goal). This reframing encourages the SLT to become comfortable with the degree of information being sought matching the perceived value and importance to the person with aphasia.

Part II: Procedural guidance

The above principles underpinning Establishing Assessment and Goal-focused Assessment are central to the success of the approach, as they influence how certain clinical skills are applied and the encounter constructed. Clinical confidence in conducting the more formal, test-based assessment activities that typically fall under Goal-focused Assessment is more likely, given the procedural instruction and analysis associated with these, often published, methods. The lack of detailed guidance for the more informal, discourse-based activity of Establishing Assessment can directly lead to lower clinical confidence and idiosyncrasy in practice. This next section therefore focuses on providing more detailed, practical guidance for the methods used in Establishing Assessment but it is by no means a step-by-step 'manual'. Where possible, readers will be signposted to more in-depth guidance available in the literature.

Informal assessment: The challenges

Defining assessment methods as informal or formal is problematic, doesn't account for the frequent combinational use of methods in practice and has the potential to diminish the SLT's expertise in applying it.

Informal methods can be defined by their lack of detailed guidance (Coelho et al., 2005), so they lend themselves to a flexible and personalized assessment encounter. However, this flexibility creates its own issue: idiosyncrasy in clinical application – in terms of why, when and how the approach is applied (process, tasks and materials) and also documented. This leads to challenges in adequately training students, newly-qualified or less experienced SLTs, as well as a shared understanding of what is being referred to in clinical discussions or documentation. *Some* degree of framework or guidance for various informal methodologies is then beneficial to address such issues.

Establishing assessment methodology

1. Semi-structured interviewing and/or conversation

The intentional use of semi-structured interviewing and/or conversation as the assessment method and context is central to Establishing Assessment. These two methods emerged as having particular value to support therapeutic assessment from our scoping review (Thomson et al., 2018) given the available guidance for rationale, timing and application of the method (compared to other informal methods).

Two protocols were identified from the scoping review for semi-structured interviewing: (1) goal-orientated conversation (in the community) using the SMARTER framework (Hersh et al. 2012), and (2) a healthcare environment-orientated conversation using the In-patient Functional Communication Interview (IFCI) (O'Halloran, Worral, Code, & Hickson, 2007). Hersh et al. (2013) clearly outline how to conduct goal-orientated semi-structured interviews using the SMARTER framework (Hersh et al., 2012). The framework leads to goal-orientated conversations being *shared, monitored, accessible, relevant, transparent, evolving* and *relationship-centred*. A case example is later presented by Hersh et al. (2013). The IFCI comprehensively outlines the information to be sought from review of medical records for use during the interview (medical, contextual, personal) and how to conduct the semi-structured interview with the provision of an interview script and an outline of 15 'communication situations', e.g., following instructions, understanding descriptions about what is happening, going to happen or has happened, or asking questions about their care.

The scoping review also found agreement for conversation-based assessment in terms of elicitation method and stimuli. The SLT typically initiates topics, usually by requesting information (e.g., 'Tell me about your stroke/interests/work'). Hesketh et al. (2008) provide an appendix showing the starter and prompt questions asked, as well as the overall structure of the conversation, e.g., '(Opener) Can you tell me about your friends and family? (Prompts) Where do your family live? Do they live near? Who do you see in a week? What about friends or neighbours?' However, less agreement was found for analysis and documentation.

The above publications from Hesketh et al. (2008), Hersh et al. (2012), Hersh et al. (2013) and O'Halloran et al. (2007), along with the recently-updated Inpatient Functional Communication Interview: Screening, Assessment, and Intervention (IFCI: SAI) (O'Halloran, Worrall, Toffolo, & Code, 2019), are highly recommended for further reading on more detailed procedural guidance to inform the carrying out of semi-structured interviewing and/or conversation-based assessment.

2. Communication behaviours of interest

During the semi-structured interview/conversation, the SLT has to actively construct and create opportunities for the person with aphasia to display relevant communication behaviours (as well as capitalizing on spontaneously arising opportunities). Sound clinical knowledge of the relevant behaviours is crucial for both a confident and comprehensive assessment. Sourcing an exhaustive account of the desired communication behaviours is outside of this chapter's scope. However, comprehensive communication performance typically includes linguistic performance across both micro (e.g., single word language tasks) and macro levels (e.g., discourse types). It is also very beneficial to consider relevant cognitive and perceptual skills involved in the respective communication activities.

Appendix I provides an example of my Establishing Assessment documentation form (used after the assessment encounter) and highlights the communication behaviours that are typically explored during my own Establishing Assessment encounter.

3. Eliciting the communication behaviours

Confidence in knowing what needs to be explored allows for efforts to focus on how best to explore and elicit the behaviours – in a manner that upholds the principles of the approach. Planning how the semi-structured interview/conversation intends to progress is helpful *prior* to the assessment encounter. Generating a template interview/conversational 'script' is helpful in this planning (with potential variations depending on severity) – see the IFCI: SAI for an example of a clinical script (O'Halloran et al., 2019). The template script will depend on several factors including the clinical setting, time since the onset of aphasia and what is known about the person with aphasia, e.g. degree of personal information or known severity (if further into their recovery).

Planning the Establishing Assessment session/script includes:

- Appropriate introduction and ending of the assessment session.

- Identifying the main topic/s, expected sub-topics and questions to be used as openers, including when and in what order the questions will be asked.

- How and when certain communication behaviours will be elicited as naturally as possible, including what supported conversation techniques (Kagan, 1998) may be required and how they can be incorporated into the activity (e.g., using written choices to explore reading ability). Confidence in supported conversation techniques can have a direct impact on the success of the interaction.

The script encourages the aim of the semi-structured interview/conversation to be made clear to the person with aphasia during the session introduction and summing up, given its apparent informal nature. The degree of explanation will vary depending on the context and severity of aphasia. The example below is adapted from the IFCI: SAI (O'Halloran et al., 2019) and is similar to the type of opener used in my own, hospital-based (stroke service), Establishing Assessment encounters:

Hello! My name is _____. I'm a speech and language therapist. Part of my job is to help you, your family/friends and hospital staff communicate as easily as possible. Sometimes this can be difficult after a stroke. I'd like to do this by having a chat with you. We can talk about what has been happening, you can ask any questions or share any worries, and we can spend some time getting to know each other. If we have any difficulty chatting, then I will see if there's anything I can do to help. Does that sound OK?

The main topic/s, sub-topics and questions used during the interview, including their order, does require some flexibility, e.g., in order to be responsive to the needs of the person with aphasia, the time point in the recovery, and their situation. However, common themes emerge in clinical encounters at any time point/situation that can guide preparation. These tend to include the patient's knowledge and experience of their health and aphasia journey to date, the impact of their health and aphasia on their daily life, how they spend their days (i.e., activities and roles), where and with whom, and their overall wellbeing. These conversational topics naturally lend themselves to sustain the focus of the semi-structured interview/conversation on what is important, i.e., their goals.

Appendix II provides an example script from my Establishing Assessment practice, outlining a sequence of questions that might typically be asked, as well as how and when certain communication behaviours can be elicited during this sequence. The behaviours are typically elicited;

1. *Either*, where the question asked corresponds and lends itself to elicitation of a particular behaviour; for example, simple instruction following can be explored during environmental set-up at the beginning of the encounter (e.g., 'do you want to sit in your chair/sit up/find your glasses?'), writing skill by asking the person to write their address when talking about where they live, or procedural description when asking the person about how they carry out a specific activity (e.g., 'can you talk me through your way of doing X'?).

2. *Or*, in response to an encountered communication challenge, where the behaviour is explored as a communication support offered by the SLT; for example, repetition, spelling to dictation or spelling aloud can be explored as a potential strategy by offering a word that couldn't be spontaneously provided (e.g., 'does it help if I say it? Can you write it if I spell it out? Does it help to say it if you read it aloud?').

The above methodology requires being comfortable with a high level of responsiveness and flexibility specifically relating to how best explore a given communication behaviour, particularly in relation to whatever naturally arises within the encounter, e.g., its co-construction. This may be capitalizing on unexpected personal information or issues that are shared (e.g., concern about finances if in hospital), unexpected activities brought into the interaction by the person with aphasia (e.g., exploring reading ability via text messages if the person brings into the interaction a mobile phone to show photos of family), or the severity of aphasia itself (e.g., much improved performance expected from medical records).

The above skills of responsiveness and flexibility are core clinical skills, familiar to every SLT, e.g., the stepping up or down of an activity, the tools available to facilitate communication. The Establishing Assessment methodology doesn't necessarily require a new skill set but does encourage a consideration of *how* certain skills and techniques are applied. This is particularly true in relation to 'testing' – a very familiar clinical methodology. The informal, discourse-based approach of Establishing Assessment requires a certain degree of vigilance in order to prevent inadvertent 'testing'. Confidence in moving away from testing in Establishing Assessment (towards testing mainly within the Goal-focused Assessment) can be supported by reflecting on what testing provides in order to consider how these aims can still be met. Two common reasons are quantification of performance and relationship to theoretical knowledge.

Establishing Assessment methodology doesn't prevent quantification, it simply alters what information might be of value to quantify, e.g., capturing how many family members' names are spoken correctly when discussing family, or how many activities of daily living are named when a person describes their daily/weekly routine. Despite quantification still being possible, the approach does perhaps allow for more clinically meaningful qualitive description of performance and its associated impact, e.g., certain information topics that are easier to understand and therefore certain conversation topics/settings that might be more problematic.

Similarly, although detailed, in-depth assessment of communication behaviours is not the intention of Establishing Assessment; it doesn't prevent performance being linked to theoretical knowledge, e.g., cognitive neuropsychological models such as Primary Systems Hypothesis (Patterson & Lambon Ralph, 1999). This model suggests that all language activities (e.g., naming, reading, and spelling) are supported by the same underlying, interconnected language system which is comprised of three core domains (semantics, phonology and orthography/vision). It implies that performance in a given task, e.g., naming, will be reflected across other language tasks, e.g., reading, comprehension or writing, depending on the degree of impairment in the three core domains and the contribution of each core domain to a given language task. For example, poor repetition ability, which is indicative of impairment to the phonological domain, suggests reduced performance will be reflected in every other language task that requires phonology (e.g., naming, spoken comprehension, reading aloud, spelling to dictation). The model helps predict performance for language activities that have not been actively explored in the assessment encounter, based on how the model suggests performance/impairment is produced. The integrity of the model's domains and routes can then be informed from early on in assessment encounter, guiding the areas and activities to explore in further assessment, and how to do so, particularly if further Goal-based Assessment is agreed.

An Establishing Assessment 'Toolkit'

Considering all of the above, it is in no way surprising that students, newly-qualified or less experienced SLTs are drawn towards more formal assessment practices or informal 'testing' where the communication behaviours of interest are clearly laid out and the 'online' moment-by-moment processing demands upon the SLT are more readily managed through specific procedural guidance (e.g., elicitation methods and documentation). Acknowledging the draw towards the more formalized practices, because of the available procedural guidance, helps inform how to support SLTs to be more confident in carrying out Establishing Assessment until familiarity is established. Confidence in carrying out Establishing Assessment can be supported by a simple 'toolkit' comprising of:

- *A recording form*: Providing a visual aide memoir of what communication behaviours to elicit or identify, as well as an accessible and consistent manner of documentation.

- *A template 'script'*: Outlining a potential structure for the more naturalistic interaction consisting of topics relevant to the timing of the encounter, the context, and the individual, as well as potential elicitation points and methods for the communication behaviours of interest.

- *(Supported) conversation resources*: Relevant to the interview/conversation topics, elicitation points and methods, e.g., pen, paper, tablet device, pictographic cards of interests/everyday activities, rating scales.

Summary

The ethos, value and structure of *Establishing Assessment* and *Goal-focused Assessment* shared in this chapter is the outcome of a personal search for a clinically satisfying approach to assessment practice. The approach aims to capitalize on, and demonstrate, the specialist skill, role and value of the SLT in supporting people with aphasia at any time point and in any setting. It centres on the SLT *re-framing* the purpose of assessment in order to consider how best to apply certain skills and tools in constructing an assessment encounter that is highly-principled, is personalized and tailored to best capture the real-life impact of aphasia, and is driven by the priorities and goals of the person with aphasia (Hinckley, 2017). This re-framing of assessment encourages the alignment of assessment practice with wider intervention practice, supporting aphasia management to be of greatest value to the person with aphasia (Worrall, 2019) from beginning to end.

References

Armstrong, E. (2000). Aphasic discourse analysis: The story so far. *Aphasiology*, 14, 875–892.

Armstrong, E. & Mortensen, L. (2006). Everyday talk: Its role in assessment and treatment for individuals with aphasia. *Brain Impairment*, 7, 175–189.

Armstrong, L., Brady, M., Mackenzie, C., & Norrie, J. (2007). Transcription-less analysis of aphasic discourse: A clinician's dream or a possibility? *Aphasiology*, 21, 355–374.

Armstrong, E., Bryant, L., Ferguson, A., & Simmons-Mackie, N. (2016). Approaches to assessment and treatment of everyday talk in aphasia. In: I. Papathanasiou & P. Coppens (Eds), *Aphasia and Related Neurogenic Communication Disorders*, 2nd edn. (pp.269–285). Burlington, MA: Jones & Bartlett Learning.

Barnes, S. & Bloch, S. (2019). Why is measuring communication difficult? A critical review of current speech pathology concepts and measures. *Clinical Linguistics & Phonetics*, 33(3), 219–236.

Beeke, S., Wilkinson, R., & Maxim, J. (2003). Exploring aphasic grammar 2: Do language testing and conversation tell a similar story? *Clinical Linguistics and Phonetics*, 17, 109–134.

Bright, F.A.S & Reeves, B. (2020). Creating therapeutic relationships through communication: A qualitative metasynthesis from the perspectives of people with communication impairment after stroke. *Disability and Rehabilitation*. doi:10.1080/09638288.2020.1849419

Bright, F., Kayes, N., Worrall, L., &McPherson, K. (2015). A conceptual review of engagement in healthcare and rehabilitation. *Disability and Rehabilitation*, 37(8), 643–654.

Bryant, L., Spencer, E., & Ferguson, A. (2016). Clinical use of linguistic discourse analysis for the assessment of language in aphasia. *Aphasiology*, 31(10), 1105–1126.

Centre for Clinical Research Excellence in Aphasia Rehabilitation (CCREIAR) (2014). *Australian Aphasia Rehabilitation Pathway and Aphasia Rehabilitation Best-practice Statements*. Available at: http://www.aphasiapathway.com.au (accessed May 2021).

Coelho, C., Ylvisaker, M., & Turkstra, L. (2005). Non-standardized assessment approaches for individuals with traumatic brain injuries. *Seminars in Speech and Language*, *26*(4), 223–241.

Davidson, B. & Worrall, L. (2000). The assessment of activity limitation in functional communication: challenges and choices. In: L. Worrall & C. Frattali (Eds), *Neurogenic Communication Disorders: A Functional Approach* (pp.312–328). New York, NY: Thieme.

Doedens, W.J. & Meteyard, L. (2018). The importance of situated language use for aphasia rehabilitation. https://doi.org/10.31234/osf.io/svwpf

Foster, A., Worrall, L., Rose, M., & O'Halloran, R. (2016). 'I do the best I can': An in-depth exploration of the aphasia management pathway in the acute hospital setting. *Disability and Rehabilitation*, 38, 1765–1779.

Herbert, R., Hickin, J., Howard, D., Osborne, F., & Best, W. (2008). Do picture-naming tests provide a valid assessment of lexical retrieval in conversation in aphasia? *Aphasiology*, *22*(2), 184–203.

Hersh, D., Wood, P., & Armstrong, E. (2017). Informal aphasia assessment, interaction and the development of the therapeutic relationship in the early period after stroke. *Aphasiology*, *32*(8), 876–901.

Hersh, D., Worrall, L., Howe, T., Sheratt, S., & Davidson, B. (2012) SMARTER goal setting in aphasia rehabilitation. *Aphasiology*, 26, 220–233.

Hersh, D., Worrall, L., O'Halloran, R., Brown, K., Grohn, B., & Rodriguez, A. (2013). Assess for success: Evidence for therapeutic assessment. In: N. Simmons-Mackie, J. King & D. Beukelman (Eds), *Supporting Communication for Adults with Acute and Chronic Aphasia* (pp. 145–164). Baltimore, MD: Paul H. Brookes.

Hesketh, A., Long, A., Patchick, E., Lee, J., & Bowen, A. (2008). The reliability of rating conversation as a measure of functional communication following stroke. *Aphasiology*, *22*, 970–984.

Hinckley, J. (2017). Selecting, combining, and bundling different therapy approaches. In: P. Coppens & J. Patterson (Eds), *Aphasia Rehabilitation: Clinical Challenges*. Burlington, MA: Jones & Bartlett.

Jaecks, P., Hielscher-Fastabend, M., &Stenneken, P. (2012). Diagnosing residual aphasia using spontaneous speech analysis. *Aphasiology*, *26*, 953–970.

Kagan, A. (1998). Supported conversation for adults with aphasia: Methods and resources for training conversation partners. *Aphasiology*, *12*, 816–830.

Kagan, A. & Simmons-Mackie, N. (2007). Beginning with the end: Outcome-driven assessment and intervention with life participation in mind. *Topics in Language Disorders*, *27*(4), 309–317.

Kelley, S. & Goldstein, H. (2019). Examining performance on a process-based assessment of word learning in relation to vocabulary knowledge and learning in vocabulary intervention. *Seminare in Speech Language, 40*(5), 344–358.

Lawton, M., Sage, K., Haddock, G., Conroy, P., & Serrant, L. (2018a). Speech and language therapists' perspectives of therapeutic alliance construction and maintenance in aphasia rehabilitation post-stroke. *International Journal of Language Communication Disorders, 53*(3), 550–563.

Lawton, M., Haddock, G., Conroy, P., Serrant, L., & Sage, K. (2018b). People with aphasia's perception of the therapeutic alliance in aphasia rehabilitation post stroke: A thematic analysis. *Aphasiology, 32*(12), 1397–1417.

Myrberg, K., Hydén, L., & Samuelsson, C. (2017). Different approaches in aphasia assessments: A comparison between test and everyday conversations. *Aphasiology, 32*(4), 417–435.

O'Halloran, R., Worrall, L., Code, C., & Hickson, L. (2007). Development of a measure of communication activity for the acute hospital setting Part II: Item analysis, selection and reliability. *Journal of Medical Speech-Language Pathology, 15*, 51–66.

O'Halloran, R., Worrall, L., Toffolo, D., & Code, C. (2019). *Inpatient Functional Communication Interview: Screening, Assessment, and Intervention.* San Diego, CA: Plural Publishing.

Patterson, K. & Lambon Ralph, M. (1999). Selective disorders of reading? *Current Opinion in Neurobiology, 9*(2) 235–239.

Pound, C. & Jensen, L. (2018). Humanising communication between nursing staff and patients with aphasia: Potential contributions of the Humanisation Values Framework. *Aphasiology, 32*(10), 1225–1249.

Ramsberger, G. & Rende, B., (2002). Measuring transactional success in the conversation of people with aphasia. *Aphasiology, 16*, 337–353.

Simmons-Mackie, N., Worrall, L., Murray, L., Enderby, P., Rose, M., Paek, E., & Klippion, A. on behalf of the Aphasia United Best Practices Working Group and Advisory Committee (2017). The top ten: Best practice recommendations for aphasia. *Aphasiology, 31*(2), 131–151.

Spreen, O. & Risser, A. (2003). *Assessment of Aphasia.* New York, NY: Oxford University Press.

Thomson, J., Gee, M., Sage, K., & Walker, T. (2018). What 'form' does informal assessment take? A scoping review of the informal assessment literature for aphasia. *International Journal of Language & Communication Disorders, 53*, 659–674.

Togher, L. (2003). Do I have green hair? 'Conversations' in aphasia therapy. In: S. Parr, J. Duchan, & C. Pound (Eds), *Aphasia Inside Out: Reflections on Communication Disability* (pp.65–79). Milton Keynes, UK: Open University Press.

World Health Organisation (WHO). (2001). *International Classification of Functioning, Disability and Health. Report.* Geneva: WHO.

Worrall, L. (2019). The seven habits of highly effective aphasia therapists: The perspective of people living with aphasia. *International Journal of Speech Language Pathology, 21*(5), 438–447.

Appendix I

APHASIA: Establishing Assessment record sheet

Patient Name: Date:

SPOKEN EXPRESSION	SPOKEN COMPREHENSION
Accurate Yes / No? **Yes / No bias?** **Naming / generation:** **Error type/s:** **Repetition:** Y/ N **Reading aloud:** Y/ N **Fluency:** *fluent / telegrammatic / non-fluent* **Speed:** **Content:** Quality – *empty / key words / rich?* Quantity – *minimal / adequate / excessive?* Formulaic? Word Ty spe? **Syntactic structure / grammar:** **Speech acts/ functions:** **Discourse type/s:** **Cohesion & Coherence:** **Strategies (Self /SLT):**	**Content word / key word understanding?** **Sentence understanding?** Type? Speech function / act? **Discourse understanding:** Conversation? Procedure? Narrative? Description? **Claims 'v' displays of understanding:** **Strategies (Self /SLT):**
SPELLING / WRITING	READING
Personal details? **Copying:** Y/ N **Naming / generation:** **Spelling to dictation / Spelling aloud:** **Error type/s:** **Content:** Word Type? Quality – *empty / key words / rich?* Quantity – *minimal / adequate / excessive?* **Syntactic structure / grammar?** **Cohesion & Coherence?** **Strategies (Self /SLT):**	**Content word / key word understanding?** **Error type/s:** **Sentence understanding?** *Type / Complexity?* **Text level understanding?** *Complexity?* **Inferencing?** **Speed?** **Strategies (Self /SLT):**

Continues overleaf

INTERACTION	COGNITION & PERCEPTION
Situational understanding?	**Orientation:** *Time, place, person*
Communicative intent & initiation?	**Recognition:**
Social cues: provision & perception?	*Person / Object / Picture / Sound*
Non-verbal expression:	**Vision?**
• *Vocalisation*	**Attention / Concentration:**
• *Facial expression*	*Fleeting / sustained / divided / fixed / distractible*
• *Nods / shakes head*	**Memory:**
• *Referential pointing*	*Working memory / recall / episodic, short /*
• *Gestures / co-speech gestures*	*long-term*
Turn taking:	**Task Comprehension?**
Minimal - fills turn only	
Progresses / sequential	**Processing speed?**
Topic maintenance & progression:	**Insight & awareness?**
Maintains / tangential	
Topic relevant shift / unable to shift / Repetitive	**Planning & sequencing?**
Repair:	**Reasoning & problem solving?**
Self-initiated / other-initiated repair	**Monitoring?**
Successful?	
Communicative competence: effective / reduced	
Communicative burden: self / other	

Environment	*Facilitators:*	*Barriers:*

Info gathered (e.g., *goals* / valued activities, socio-biographic):

STRENGTHS: DIFFICULTIES:

SUCCESSFUL STRATEGIES: NEXT STEPS:

Appendix II

Example of semi-structured interview 'template script' (hospital context), elicitation points and methods

KEY * = potential elicitation points via communication support

( ) = potential communication supports

Stages	Example script and elicitation points / methods of communication behaviours	Communication behaviours/areas of interest
Introductions	*Remind you of my name...* **(SLT says and write name)** *Before we get going – can I check what you would prefer me to call you?* If not able to name: **Can you write it?* **(offer pen, support as needed, e.g., initial letter, copy)** **Let me write some options for you to choose...* **(Support: written list of name shortenings / surname)** **Can you read it aloud? / Does it help to say it after me?*	- Pragmatics, e.g., social cues - Naming Personal single written naming Personal single word reading Reading aloud / repetition
Environment	*And just to make sure that you are comfortable as well:* *- e.g., sit up / sit in this chair* *- e.g., clear the table* *- e.g., move the drink* *And do you need any glasses / hearing aid?* **(*Support as needed: visual cues, e.g., referential pointing, gesture...)**	- Spoken comprehension, e.g., simple commands

Continues overleaf

Orientation	*It's helpful to make sure you know where we are and what is happening at the moment.* *Do you know where we are at the moment?* If not able to name: **Can you write it?* **(offer pen, support as needed)** **Let me write some options for you to choose…* **(Support: written option of places / list of local hospitals)** **Can you read it aloud? / Does it help to say it after me?* *Do you know what's happened to you / why you came to hospital? What have the doctors said? How are you feeling? What's is different at the moment / What are you having difficulty with? How are these problems affecting what you can to / take part in…? Is that a problem…?* **Support as needed: "Can you write anything to help tell me…or show me… or draw…or if I write some options for you to read…use this scale…"*	- Naming single written naming single word reading reading aloud / repetition - Spoken comprehension, e.g., questions - Spoken expression, e.g., situational narrative / info sharing (Use of additional means, e.g., gestures, drawing, rating scales, etc., spelling and reading)
Information provision Wellbeing	Explanation about current situation / communication diagnoses as required / what to expect re: hospital stay… **Support as needed: visual supports, e.g., drawing to help provide information needed to pt / images / videos* *Do you want to check anything I have explained? Have any questions about what's happening?* **Support as needed* *Are you worried or concerned about anything at the moment?* **Support as needed* *How are your feelings at the moment? (* Support as needed, e.g., written choices / drawings of different emotions)*	- Spoken comprehension, e.g., info exchange / situational narrative - Spoken expression, e.g., asking questions (Response to additional means, etc)

Information gathering/ Goals	*The hospital staff are going to work with you and your family to try and help you get ready to leave hospital at the right time. It's helpful for us to get to know more about what life is like at home / before hospital / what is important to you. Can I ask you about that?*	- Spoken comprehension, e.g., personal, sociobiographic questions
Home	*Where do you live? Can you write your address?* ***If not able to name/write: Support as needed, e.g., local map, written choices, written copy, reading aloud / repetition**	- Personal naming and spelling
Family	*Does anyone live with you? Have you any children / grandchildren? Tell me more about them…How often do you see / how keep in touch / what do you do together / do for each other / how well do you get along? Are you worried or concerned about your family at the moment?* **Support as needed, e.g., written choices, drawings, offer pen for spelling**	-Spoken expression e.g. narrative, personal, procedural, descriptive discourse
Activities and daily living Goals	*And looking after yourself at home – what jobs do you have to do at home / who does the jobs at home / do you have any help at home, e.g.* • *Cooking? (e.g., What's your favourite dish, can you tell me about cooking your favourite dish…)* • *Cleaning? (e.g. Tell me about what you have to do…)* • *Manages the money? (e.g., Which bank do you use, bills you have, etc.)* • *Shopping? (e.g.m Which supermarket do you go to? How often do you go? How do you go?)* • *Driving? (e.g., What kind of car have you got? How often do you use it?)* • *Gardening (e.g., what do you grow, your gardening jobs)* • *DIY?* ***Support as needed: e.g., offer pen for spelling, drawing, provide written choices, household activity picture cards sorting (e.g., sorting to patient's / partner name)**	- Spoken expression, e.g., narrative, personal, procedural, descriptive discourse
Goals	*What does the routine of your day or week look like? Tell me more about…* ***Support as needed: e.g., creating a day or week overview / timetable, e.g., writing / placing written options / drawings into corresponding time or day slot** *Are you worried or concerned about anything at home at the moment? Are you worried or concerned about being able to do any of these activities at the moment? Would you want to focus on any of them whilst in hospital?* *** Support as needed…**	- Spoken expression, e.g., narrative, personal, procedural, descriptive discourse

Continues overleaf

Interests / goals	*What about time for yourself / how do you like to spend your free time / what do you enjoy / what are your interests?* ***Support as needed: e.g., offer pen for spelling / drawing, providing written choices, Interest activity picture cards sorting likes / dislikes*** *Are you worried or concerned about being able to do any of these activities at the moment? Are any of them important to focus on whilst in hospital?* **Support as needed…**	- Personal narrative / sequence description
Confirmation Communica- tion summary / actions Closing	*Thank you for telling me lots about you there, and what life is like for you. It helps us know what is important to you / what to work on / what you are worried about…* *Whilst we were talking, I noticed…* (SLT explanation of strengths / difficulties / communication supports) *Share with staff and your family…* *Talk more next time / come and see you again…*	- Pragmatics, e.g., social cues, ending the interaction

3 Rebuilding a life with aphasia: Listening to what is important using Solution Focused Brief Therapy

Sarah Northcott, John Smejka and Paula Smejka

Many people with aphasia describe a profound sense of loss. This chapter explores the psychosocial impact of living with aphasia, the role of the Speech and Language Therapist, and outlines one specific therapy approach: Solution Focused Brief Therapy (SFBT). Key aspects of SFBT are illustrated using a case example. The chapter also includes a first-hand account of living with aphasia and receiving SFBT, as well as a spouse's perspective on loss and change.

Why should Speech and Language Therapists consider the emotional wellbeing of people with aphasia?

Having a stroke and aphasia challenges a person's assumptions about their life, their sense of who they are, their hopes and plans for the future. The social and emotional impact of aphasia can be considerable. People living with aphasia have been found to have less contact with friends and are involved in fewer social activities (Cruice, Worrall, & Hickson, 2006; Hilari & Northcott, 2006). Aphasia is a stronger predictor of having a weakened social network six months post-stroke than severity of stroke or disability (Northcott, Marshall, & Hilari, 2016). Further, feeling isolated is closely linked to low mood (Hilari et al., 2010; Northcott, Moss, Harrison, & Hilari, 2016). Around 31% of people are depressed following a stroke (Hackett & Pickles, 2014) and this figure is higher for those with aphasia. One study reported that 70% of people with aphasia at 3 months and 62% at 12 months post-stroke fulfilled the DSM-III-R criteria for depression (Kauhanen et al., 2000). Expressive communication impairment has also been found to be a significant predictor of depression at one- and six-months post-stroke (Thomas & Lincoln, 2008). A stroke takes its toll on the whole family. Family members describe having to take on new roles and responsibilities, which can leave them feeling exhausted and lonely (Winkler, Bedford, Northcott, & Hilari, 2014).

UK Stroke Guidelines state that the same importance should be given to addressing the psychological as to the physical consequences of stroke (NHS Improvement, 2011). In terms of the role of the Speech and Language Therapist (SLT) there has been increasing recognition that communication and language does not happen in a vacuum, but is intricately woven into a person's social relationships, identity and participation in life. Thus, through taking a more holistic approach it may be more possible to achieve communication goals. This is reflected in professional guidelines. The UK Royal College of Speech and Language Therapists (2005, p.98) states that therapists should "address emotional health and enable participation in an individual's social context". Similarly, the American Speech-Language-Hearing Association (2016) states that the SLT role includes "counselling interactions related to emotional reactions, thoughts, feelings and behaviours that result from living with the communication disorder". Practising SLTs overwhelmingly agree that addressing psychological wellbeing is part of their role: 98% of Australian SLTs (Sekhon, Douglas, & Rose, 2015) and 93% of UK SLTs (Northcott, Simpson, Moss, Ahmed, & Hilari, 2017). Yet these surveys also found that only a minority of SLTs felt confident in this area: 31% of Australian SLTs and 42% of UK SLTs. A main barrier cited in both surveys was that SLTs perceived themselves to be underskilled. Other barriers included lack of time, caseload pressures, and lack of ongoing specialist support.

UK Stroke Guidelines (NHS Improvement, 2011) recommend a collaborative model of care. For low-level mood problems, it is suggested that psychological care is the responsibility of the whole stroke team, and potentially may be addressed through active listening and providing advice and information. For mild-to-moderate mood problems, guidelines suggest that clinical psychologists should support stroke specialist staff, such as SLTs, to address the psychological needs of the person post-stroke. For severe and persistent mood problems, people should be seen by a clinical psychologist or psychiatrist. Yet a Stroke Association survey found that less than half of English stroke units had access to psychology services, and only 20% of people post-stroke felt they were given information, advice and support in coping with the emotional aspects of having a stroke (Stroke Association, 2015).

There are additional concerns for people with aphasia as there is variation in how confident and skilled mental health professionals are when working with this client group (Baker, Worrall, Rose, & Ryan, 2019; Northcott, Simpson, Moss, Ahmed, & Hilari, 2017). In particular, people with more marked aphasia are reported to find accessing appropriate mental health services challenging (Northcott et al., 2018). A further concern is that the current evidence base for effective psychological therapies for people with aphasia is limited (Baker et al., 2017): people with aphasia are often excluded from psychological stroke research due to their language disability.

A Christmas Stroke

By John Smejka

I was 54 when I suffered a stroke. Christmas Eve 2011 I went out with my buddy of 50 years for a Christmas drink. I said to Graham I've got splitting headache, so I called the taxi and he drove me home. Christmas Day I woke up with the same headache and also I couldn't see through my left eye. So I drove myself to the Lincoln Hospital, it was about 6am in morning. I called Paula on the phone and she met me there. At the hospital I said think it's a problem with my eyes. The Lincoln hospital said we haven't got eye specialist, they are on leave, so we went to Boston hospital, it was about 30 miles away. It was about 4pm the stroke hit me. I lost my feelings on the right side, leg, arms, and the left eye has gone. And also my speech was gone.

Straight after my stroke I was unable to converse at all. I had my basic needs to trial and error. There was a laminate on my table which said yes and no and there was pictures so I could point to them. I was 'released' in about 9 weeks. I came home with a wheelchair.

I am still an intelligent man

Words finally came (slowly). I am lucky in that I understand about 99% of what is said to me. I would say that about 99% reading. I am able to write about 15%. Then about 5% of speech.

I am still an intelligent man, I got a BSc and MSc. My thoughts, ideas, feelings haven't changed, is just the fact information going in, normal speed, but information going out – slow, slow speed. When I meet people on the street I can greet them (hello, good morning, hiya) but if they stop that is hard for me. I can think of what to say but it takes long time to say it.

What the difference now, well

I can't work anymore. I was the Head of Engineering for Anglian Water, I think it's about 75% was talking and about 25% writing. I loved work, I worked 12 hours a day. Now I have retired. Friends: I had a large circle of friends. Today is only three friends. I got an IPad for reading/ writing/ emails/ Skype/ FaceTime. I am able read newspapers and magazines. Before my stroke I didn't read books at all in leisure time I was doing other things like: Paula, kids, Gym, Swim, Sauna, Walk, Friends, Guitar (those were the days) but now I estimate that I read about 30 books year.

Kids. I have got 4 children, Emily, Tom, Andy and Rosie. The kids have grown up. But I should have spent more time with them.

Paula: We were engaged for ten weeks before my stroke. We had so, so many plans.

A wife's perspective on loss and change

By Paula Smejka

It is impossible to put into words how stroke changed our life. Before the stroke, John was an amazing communicator; he told stories that made us laugh; he gave advice that was sensible and well thought through; he could tell me in dozens of different ways why he loved me.

In the early days after the stroke, our focus was on any communication at all, we celebrated 'yes' and 'no', we worked for hours on every exercise ever suggested. John did improve – short conversations require patience and perseverance but are possible. But the frivolous doesn't happen; the words he used to have to bring me down from a temper don't exist; the encouragement and reassurance that things will be alright isn't backed up with language.

I look at how our life has changed, our life as individuals, as a couple, as a family and I realise how lonely and isolated we have become. We rarely see friends any more. The difficulties around access and planning, the challenges with communication, they are there every day, in everything we do, and I understand that this makes spending time with us hard. Other people only have to live with these difficulties in the hours they spend with John. But John has to live with this every minute of every day for the rest of his life. There is a sadness that stretches beyond words.

Solution Focused Brief Therapy

The remainder of this chapter describes one particular psychological therapy approach, Solution Focused Brief Therapy (SFBT). The origins of SFBT date back to the early 1980s and the Brief Family Therapy Centre in Milwaukee, USA, where Steve de Shazer, Insoo Kim Berg and colleagues explored how best to facilitate change in people's lives. They observed that there were often exceptions to patterns of problem behaviour, times when the problem was less apparent or even absent. Therapy time spent exploring these exceptions appeared to enable clients to notice possible solutions for moving forward. This focus on what the client is already doing that works became one of the central tenets of SFBT. Another development was that the work increasingly focused on the client's hopes for the future rather than problems in their past. As a consequence of this shift, they noticed that the number of sessions decreased (Ratner, George, & Iveson, 2012).

Since its conception in the 1980s, SFBT has continued to evolve and different versions of SFBT have emerged to suit varied contexts (e.g., working with people with intellectual disabilities; at-risk families; business coaching). One core assumption within SFBT is that "clients have the resources to help themselves, and that the practitioner helps them uncover, nurture and use these resources as effectively as possible" (Burns, 2016, p.155). The therapist seeks to facilitate the client in finding their own way forward, and refrains from offering advice or solutions, or making assumptions about therapy goals. The therapy typically explores a person's hopes for the future, as well as noticing what is already going well. The approach can be described as a particular way of listening: listening with a curious, not-knowing stance; listening to what is important to the client; listening to notice the building blocks that may help a person navigate their way forwards.

The strongest evidence for the effectiveness of SFBT is when working with adults who have depression (Gingerich & Peterson, 2013). When used in medical settings, a meta-analysis found it was an effective approach for achieving positive psychosocial outcomes (d=0.34, p<0.05) (Zhang, Franklin, Currin-McCulloch, Park, & Kim, 2018). It has also been shown to be flexible enough to be adapted for client groups who have limited language, such as those with a learning disability (Carrick & Randle-Phillips, 2018).

Within a stroke context, a trial reported improved mood and lower anxiety for the group that received 10 SFBT sessions shortly after hospital discharge compared with the group that received usual care, although this research excluded people with aphasia (Wichowicz, Puchalska, Rybak-Korneluk, Gąsecki, & Wiśniewska, 2017). An aphasia-accessible version of SFBT has recently been tested in the Solution Focused Brief Therapy In post-stroke Aphasia feasibility trial (SOFIA study) (Northcott et al., 2019). The trial recruited 32 people with aphasia and employed a wait-list design. Participants received up to six therapy sessions, spaced over three months. This research found that the approach was highly acceptable, and that it was possible to adapt it to be accessible even to those with severe aphasia (Northcott, Simpson et al., 2021). In the SOFIA trial, the intervention was delivered by SLTs, giving encouragement that it is feasible for SLTs to deliver SFBT providing they have appropriate training and ongoing support. The approach lends itself to being integrated with discipline-specific work (Burns, 2016). It is possible to draw on the core assumptions or use some of the solution-focused questions or techniques, and blend these with existing speech and language therapy skills and knowledge. SLTs have described it as a holistic framework facilitating person-centred interactions (Northcott et al., 2018).

An illustrative case example to explore key aspects of SFBT

Joyce took part in the SOFIA study, receiving six therapy sessions over a 3-month period (Northcott et al., 2019). She had her stroke about five years previously. Although she scored as having mild aphasia on the Frenchay Aphasia Screening Test (Enderby, Wood, & Wade, 1987), she experienced her aphasia as distressing and frustrating. Given her low mood, Joyce was also supported to seek advice from her GP. All identifying details have been changed and a pseudonym used.

Establishing best hopes

In a first session a Solution Focused therapist will seek to find out what is important to a person, and what they are hoping for from the therapy. The client is considered the expert in their own lives: it is for them to know what will make a meaningful difference to them. A typical question to elicit a focus for the therapy might be: 'What are your best hopes from our talking together?'

When Joyce was asked about her best hopes from the therapy, she said she wanted to feel happy. The therapist sought to enable Joyce to translate this 'feeling state' to observable actions. She therefore invited Joyce to describe the everyday details that would show she was feeling happy, how she would 'do' happiness. She asked Joyce what would be different if she were feeling happy. Joyce explained she would be enjoying her life, she would be giggling and laughing with others, she would be seeing friends again. This formed the basis of the 'contract' for the therapy.

'Best hopes' questions: Finding a meaningful focus for therapy

What are your best hopes from our working together?

What are you hoping for from therapy?

How will you know this has been useful? What would make the therapy worthwhile?

Helpful follow-up questions

What difference would that make to you?

What are you hoping that would lead to?

What would tell you that you were feeling X?

So instead of X, what would you like to be (feeling/doing)?

Exploring a preferred future

Having established what a client is hoping for from therapy, a Solution Focused therapist will often invite the client to describe their preferred future: what their life would look like if they achieved their 'best hopes'. The process of describing this future is argued to lend a sense of possibility to a client. The more detailed and vivid the description, the more powerful the process can be. Ratner et al. (2012) suggest a preferred future should include small concrete details rather than a description of feeling states. The focus is on what is wanted, rather than what they do not want (e.g., what will they be doing at breakfast *instead* of shouting at their children?). Often a therapist will ask 'interactional' questions: what others will notice about the client. This is another way to make inner feelings more visible and translate them into small observable actions.

The therapist invited Joyce to imagine waking up tomorrow feeling happy, enjoying life. What was the first thing she would notice? Joyce was encouraged to describe the breakfast scene. She said she would be singing badly as she made a cup of tea, would notice people walking outside, and think: I want to be them, outside, in life. Her description of 'tomorrow' evolved to include what her husband and son would notice about her that would tell them she was enjoying life. She imagined how she and her husband would go into town, how they would window shop and look at the billboards for shows, with takeaway hot chocolates.

These descriptions open up small, detailed possibilities for the client; it is up to the client which aspects of the description they take away and use in their life. As such the conversation is not used as a way for the therapist to set specific goals.

Preferred future questions

Suppose tomorrow you find a way to be [insert best hope]. What's the first thing you'll notice?

Imagine tomorrow is a really good day. How will you know it's going well?

What will be first sign you're moving in the right direction?

Useful follow up questions

Who else will notice? How will your [husband] know you are feeling [insert best hope]?

What else? (useful question to elicit further details)

Exploring what is already working – use of scaling questions

A key aspect of SFBT is enabling clients to notice their own strategies and what is already working. One tool is a scale, going from 0 to 10. Typically, a therapist may place the 'best hope' at 10, and the opposite at 0. The scale, however, can be used flexibly. At 10, a therapist may choose 'living with aphasia as well as anyone', or 'handling my aphasia'. The client is then invited to place themselves on the scale. A therapist is likely first to acknowledge where the client has placed themselves, and notice any distress associated with their answer. Once they gauge the client feels sufficiently heard, the scale can be used to explore what is already working. If, for example, someone places themselves at a 3/10, the therapist would explore with them how come 3 and not lower. This is one way of enabling people to name and accord significance to all that they are already doing that is helpful to them. A therapist may then choose to spend time exploring how they would know they were one point up the scale. Again, the emphasis of this conversation is not establishing specific goals for the client, rather, it is to enable a client to visualize how moving forwards might look.

In Joyce's case, in the first session '10' on her scale was 'happiness/enjoying life'. She placed herself at a 2/10. The therapist followed up by asking her where she was on this scale a month earlier, which she had described as a particular low point. She placed herself at 0/10. The therapist gave her space to share her feelings of profound pain. They then explored how she had managed to move from 0 to 2. It took encouragement and support for Joyce to start noticing her own small steps and the resources that she had drawn on to manage this shift, despite feeling very low. She explained that yesterday she had been able to set herself a small task and carry it out: she had bought two Christmas presents. Over the last week, she had also started to plan a holiday in the mountains in the Spring with her husband. On reflection, these two acts gave her hope.

Scaling questions

On a scale of 0-10, where 10 is [insert relevant word or phrase, e.g., handling the stroke], and 0 is the opposite, where are you now?

How come 3, and not lower?

If you moved up one point, how would you know?

Noticing what is going well

A core part of the therapist's role is to enable their client to become more aware of their own skills and resources. There is a belief that strategies and 'solutions' that are embedded within the client's life are more likely to be sustainable than solutions imposed on them.

In Joyce's case, follow-up sessions tended to start with the therapist asking Joyce what she had been pleased to notice since the previous session. The therapist would often list these, writing down key words. The therapist sometimes chose to amplify, by inviting Joyce to notice how she had managed to achieve something, what it told her about herself, who else had noticed, what difference it made to her. Joyce described myriad details of everyday life that were small signs to her that she was moving in her preferred direction: hoovering the whole flat, unloading the dishwasher, looking after her son's cat, starting to cook again. Many of her 'signs of progress' involved her family and shifts within family relationships. She described everyday interactions with her husband and son, and the activities they were starting to do together again (going to a local market, a meal out at a restaurant, a night away). She started to care about her appearance again and took pleasure in clothes shopping for the first time since her stroke. In her final session, she shared that she was now talking with strangers. Previously she had lacked confidence due to her aphasia. She explained to the therapist that she thought differently now. Instead of worrying about her aphasia, she reasoned: 'why not?' and just did it. She described how she started a conversation with a stranger in a lift, talking about clothes. This had made her feel good about herself. She told the therapist she was 'going out with a smile', and when she smiled, others smiled back. She said she was feeling happy again.

Some of these 'signs of progress' related to her initial description of her preferred future, but many did not. The therapist's role is to enable the person to notice and give significance to all that they are doing that is enabling them to move forwards in their preferred direction.

Celebrating achievements

What have you been pleased to notice?

What have you been proud of?

What's been going in the right direction?

Instances of success

When are the times that it goes a bit better?

Tell me about times when you [feel happier/ calmer]?

Balancing acknowledgement and possibility

It has been said that a Solution Focused practitioner will have one foot in possibility, one foot in acknowledgement (O'Hanlon & Beadle, 1996). A person needs to feel heard, to feel their situation and experiences have been understood, that their distress has been witnessed by the therapist. As such, the therapist will not minimize or dismiss their distress, or move into future-focused conversations too quickly. While the Solution Focused therapist will be listening out for the hints of light in a person's story, they will also give the person the space they need to share darker emotions.

Joyce described how she used to be a chatty person: she felt the aphasia had taken this from her. The stroke and aphasia also meant she had to give up a job which she loved. She described traumatic experiences associated with the aphasia, for example an occasion when she could not get home because she was unable to say her address. She also described other losses: friends moving away, bereavement, family illness. She explained she had tried to 'be strong' and shield others from how disorientated and sad she was feeling. Unable to keep this up, she sank into depression, no longer interested in anything or anyone.

The therapist gave Joyce space to talk this over, listened carefully and sincerely to her account. It can be challenging to sense when a client is 'ready' to shift the conversation to considering resources or future possibilities. The therapist explored with Joyce how she had started the process of healing and recovery. The therapist also invited Joyce to reflect on her own resources which had enabled her to cope and survive her blackest moments. Through these conversations, the therapist was able to gently open up a space for Joyce to reflect on how she wanted to move forwards.

Adapting Solution Focused Brief Therapy for someone with aphasia

SBFT typically uses complex linguistic structures. It is helpful to consider how to convert typical SFBT questions to simpler forms that will match the receptive abilities of the person with aphasia. An example is exploring someone's preferred future. A classic wording for a 'preferred future' question might be: 'Imagine that overnight your best hopes from coming here to therapy were achieved, what would be different in your life tomorrow that would tell you this change had happened?' A simpler version might be: *'Tomorrow...* suppose it's a *good day*. What's different?' This may need to be further scaffolded by writing down 'tomorrow' and 'good day', referencing the client's diary to support understanding of the temporal dimension, or perhaps mapping out a 'typical day' on a timeline first with pictorial supports before introducing the concept of the preferred future.

For people with more severe aphasia, or cognitive difficulties, it can be helpful to focus on aspects of the approach that are more visual and simpler to understand, such as scaling questions, or listing what is going well, potentially with pictorial support. Scaling questions can be supported through drawing the scale out, anchoring the scale with happy/sad faces at either end, and writing a key word or drawing the key concept above the scale. Capitalizing on what the person is already comfortable with can be helpful, for example encouraging someone to share photos on their smartphone with the therapist.

SFBT celebrates a person's successful strategies. Inviting a client with aphasia to notice what strategies they already use is a way of introducing a conversation around total communication which respects the client's expertise. The therapist will learn from the person with aphasia how they can best support the person in accessing therapeutic conversations.

Solution Focused Brief Therapy: What's my history of me, and what is life now

By John Smejka

I was contacted by Sarah Northcott to see if wanted to join her research. So I said yes. We met at Peterborough at Paula's parents' house. It was midway London and Lincoln. We got started. Sarah ask me what's my history of me. And then, what is life now.

Paula had an idea to keep write notes so I can see what have I done. So I did. I told Sarah:

- First of all I could make myself breakfast, oat so simple.... One handed (well while I used my teeth)
- Mowing the lawn (then it was a few stripes.....now it's the whole lawn)
- Shower and dress myself
- Have a conversation with neighbour/strangers
- Walk (we did the long walk about mile)
- Agree to the ball
- Ordered my meal in Frankie and Bennies
- Good sentences
- Walk/swim/sauna/weights/cross trainer at gym
- Fixed the shovel

- Chopped wood

- Cooked chicken supreme

- Cafe alone

- Fence painting

- Hoover up, steam cleaned the bathroom

- Took my watch off and put it on again

Lot of things. I kept up for 3 months, there was about 5 things each day. Things I was pleased. Things I told Sarah. It doesn't sounds much, but was a start.

Integrating SFBT into clinical services

The core beliefs of SFBT can potentially shape all clinical interactions: the belief that the client is the expert in their own lives, not making assumptions about what is important to someone, listening out for a client's resources, building on what is already working, using the client's language and frames of reference, enabling someone to feel heard. The approach can be considered more of a mindset or a framework than a set of techniques. Nonetheless, in this chapter we have described various 'tools' or techniques, such as ways to explore with clients their goals, inviting clients to imagine their preferred future, or using scales to elicit strengths and instances of success. These tools can be borrowed and used within sessions as appropriate. As such, it is not necessary to do a discrete 'block' of SFBT to use a certain technique or solution-focused question interleaved within other therapy activities.

Another consideration is finding a way of using SFBT that sits well with the therapist. There is no one 'right' way of practising SFBT. Some questions will fit better with the therapist than others. The approach is flexible enough to be used in brief medical consultations (Sung, Mayo, & Witting, 2018), within 10-minute supervision sessions with students (Burns, 2016), working alongside a client with learning disabilities while gardening together (Bliss & Bray, 2009). There is a strong tradition of taking SFBT 'out from the therapy room, and into soup kitchens and streets' (Ratner et al., 2012, p.16): the core assumptions have been shown to translate into multiple settings. Within SLT, a therapist may begin a conversation with someone they meet on the acute stroke ward by asking: 'How can I be useful?' or 'What would be useful to you?' They may ask the client and their family what progress they've noticed the person has already made since the stroke, and ask them to look out for further progress. When goal setting at the start of a block of therapy, a therapist may ask: 'What would make these sessions worthwhile?' An SLT working on word-finding strategies might explore what difference it will make when the person with aphasia is more fluent, or times when they noticed themselves using the target words in conversation, or explore situations when conversations go better.

Another question clinicians sometimes ask is: who is this approach suitable for? Clearly, it is more straightforward to use SFBT with people who have mild aphasia. However, the SOFIA study demonstrated that it is possible to use SFBT with people who have severe aphasia, and that they were highly positive about receiving the therapy (Northcott, Simpson et al., 2021). While aspects of the approach may work less well when someone has severe aphasia (e.g., future focused description), other parts were perceived as helpful (e.g., exploring a person's resources and achievements). Speech and Language Therapists have described using SFBT in acute as well as community services (Northcott et al., 2018). Within SOFIA, the participants who appeared to gain the most from receiving a block of Solution Focused Therapy were those who had low-to-average wellbeing. SOFIA therapists perceived that the participants who made most change were those who felt stuck or at a low ebb or were wanting to make change (Northcott, Thomas et al., 2021). People with severe cognitive impairments were not included within SOFIA, nor did anyone take part who had significantly reduced insight.

A further concern for all healthcare professionals is: can this approach do harm? SFBT does not seek to uncover past difficulties or traumas, and the client is the expert and in control of the content of sessions, which arguably reduces the likelihood of causing harm. Nonetheless, SFBT questions can potentially be used to shape conversations in an unduly positive way, depriving someone of the space to share their concerns: we would urge clinicians to be mindful of this possibility, and really listen to what is important to the client, including listening to distress. Clinicians also carry a duty of care to patients: SFBT is not a risk assessment tool. Solution-focused practitioners sometimes talk about taking their 'solution-focused hat' off for a portion of a session, while they assess risk or provide expert guidance and advice. Nonetheless, it can still be helpful to interleave this advice-giving role with a listening ear for the patient's expertise, for example exploring how they might incorporate advice into their lives, or how it fits with their priorities and lived experience.

A further consideration is that in opening up conversations using solution-focused questions, clients can start to disclose concerns. SLTs can feel nervous that they may feel 'out of their depth' (Northcott et al., 2018). Really hearing someone's distress is not emotionally easy for the therapist (Simmons-Mackie & Damico, 2011). Within the SOFIA trial, the therapists highly valued not only the initial training but the ongoing specialist supervision, peer support, and being able to access real-time support when they had concerns (Northcott, Thomas et al., 2021). Similarly, in a study looking at how social workers found applying brief training in SFBT within their work, it helped having peer and organizational support (Smith, 2011). More generally, to address emotional wellbeing of people with aphasia, SLTs have described the value of working in a team with a holistic ethos, to receive support in supervision and from peers, to be able to access specialist help, for example, from a clinical psychologist, and be able to refer on or work collaboratively when they had concerns (Northcott et al., 2018). While psychological care is the responsibility of the whole stroke team, where a client has a severe or persistent mood disorder they should be seen by a psychiatrist or clinical psychologist (Kneebone, 2016). It is important SLTs do not feel on their own when addressing the psychosocial wellbeing of their clients.

Final word

It is a privilege to work with people after their stroke, to learn what really matters to them, and to be a small part of their story moving forwards. SLTs are often the first healthcare professional to enable the person with aphasia to describe their experiences and express their feelings post-stroke. They arguably have a key role to play in addressing psychological wellbeing, either through developing and nurturing their own skills, or through working collaboratively with mental health professionals and the wider team.

SFBT is not a magic wand: it cannot take away the aphasia, nor can it take away the reality that living with this new normal can be profoundly painful. Yet having the chance to share with someone else what it is like to live with the aphasia can make a real difference.

We interviewed 30 people with aphasia who had received SFBT within the SOFIA study (Northcott, Simpson et al., 2021). They valued being facilitated to notice their personal qualities and achievements, being able to explore their hopes, share their experiences and feelings, as well as the companionship and connection they felt with the therapist. Ultimately, they spoke about feeling noticed and valued as people.

Three core assumptions for therapists

SFBT is underpinned by certain core assumptions. We argue these assumptions are a humane way of approaching any therapeutic interaction. Three key assumptions are:

The client is the expert in their own life: it is for them to know how they would like their life to be, and what therapy outcome would be meaningful to them.

All clients have resources, talents, competencies, strengths and skills, even if they are not yet aware of them.

In order to create a context where change can occur, the therapist needs to hear and validate the client's experiences.

References

American Speech-Language-Hearing Association. (2016). Scope of practice in Speech-Language Pathology [Scope of Practice].

Baker, C., Worrall, L., Rose, M., Hudson, K., Ryan, B., & O'Byrne, L. (2017). A systematic review of rehabilitation interventions to prevent and treat depression in post-stroke aphasia. *Disability and Rehabilitation, 40*(16), 1780-1892. doi:10.1080/09638288.2017.1315181

Baker, C., Worrall, L., Rose, M., & Ryan, B. (2019). Stroke health professionals' management of depression after post-stroke aphasia: a qualitative study. *Disability and Rehabilitation, 43*(2), 217-228. doi:10.1080/09638288.2019.1621394

Bliss, E.V. & Bray, D. (2009). The smallest solution focused particles: Towards a minimalist definition of when therapy is solution focused. *Journal of Systemic Therapies, 28*(2), 62-74.

Burns, K. (2016). *Focus on Solutions: A Health Professional's Guide*, Revised 2nd ed. Gloucester: Solutions Books.

Carrick, H. & Randle-Phillips, C. (2018). Solution-focused approaches in the context of people with intellectual disabilities: A critical review. *Journal of Mental Health Research in Intellectual Disabilities, 11*(1), 30-53.

Cruice, M., Worrall, L., & Hickson, L. (2006). Quantifying aphasic people's social lives in the context of non-aphasic peers. *Aphasiology, 17*(4), 333-353. doi:10.1080/02687030600790136

Enderby, P., Wood, V., & Wade, D. (1987). *Frenchay Aphasia Screening Test.* Windsor UK: NFEW-Nelson.

Gingerich, W.J. & Peterson, L. (2013). Effectiveness of solution-focused brief therapy: A systematic qualitative review of controlled outcome studies. *Research on Social Work Practice*, 23(3), 266-283.

Hackett, M.L. & Pickles, K. (2014). Part I: Frequency of depression after stroke: An updated systematic review and meta-analysis of observational studies. *International Journal of Stroke*, 9(8), 1017-1025. doi:10.1111/ijs.12357

Hilari, K. & Northcott, S. (2006). Social support in people with chronic aphasia. *Aphasiology*, 20, 17-36.

Hilari, K., Northcott, S., Roy, P., Marshall, J., Wiggins, R.D., Chataway, J., & Ames, D. (2010). Psychological distress after stroke and aphasia: The first six months. *Clinical Rehabilitation*, 24(2), 181-190. doi:10.1177/0269215509346090

Kauhanen, M.L., Korpelainen, J.T., Hiltunen, P., Maatta, R., Mononen, H., Brusin, E., . . . Myllyla, V.V. (2000). Aphasia, depression, and non-verbal cognitive impairment in ischaemic stroke. *Cerebrovascular Diseases*, 10(6), 455-461. Retrieved from http://www.ncbi.nlm.nih.gov/pubmed/11070376

Kneebone, I.I. (2016). Stepped psychological care after stroke. *Disability and Rehabilitation*, 38(18), 1836-1843.

NHS Improvement. (2011). Psychological care after stroke: improving stroke services for people with cognitive and mood disorders. Accessed in http://www.nice.org.uk/

Northcott, S., Marshall, J., & Hilari, K. (2016). What factors predict who will have a strong social network following a stroke? *Journal of Speech, Language and Hearing Research*, 59(4), 772-783. doi:10.1044/2016_JSLHR-L-15-0201

Northcott, S., Moss, B., Harrison, K., & Hilari, K. (2016). A systematic review of the impact of stroke on social support and social networks: Associated factors and patterns of change. *Clinical Rehabilitation*, 30(8), 811-831.

Northcott, S., Simpson, A., Moss, B., Ahmed, N., & Hilari, K. (2017). How do Speech and Language Therapists address the psychosocial well-being of people with aphasia? Results of a UK on-line survey *International Journal of Language and Communication Disorders*, 52(3), 356-373. doi:10.1111/1460-6984.12278

Northcott, S., Simpson, A., Moss, B., Ahmed, N., & Hilari, K. (2018). Supporting people with aphasia to 'settle into a new way to be': Speech and language therapists' views on providing psychosocial support. *International Journal of Language and Communication Disorders*, 53(1), 16-29.

Northcott, S., Simpson, A., Thomas, S., Barnard, R., Burns, K., Hirani, S.P., & Hilari, K. (2021). "Now I Am Myself": Exploring how people with poststroke aphasia experienced Solution-Focused Brief Therapy within the SOFIA Trial. *Qualitative Health Research*, 31(11), 2041-2055. https://doi.org/10.1177/10497323211020290

Northcott, S., Simpson, A., Thomas, S., Hirani, S.P., Flood, C., & Hilari, K. (2019). SOlution Focused brief therapy In post-stroke Aphasia (SOFIA Trial): Protocol for a feasibility randomised controlled trial. *AMRC Open Research*, 1(11). doi:https://doi.org/10.12688/amrcopenres.12873.2

Northcott, S., Thomas, S., James, K., Simpson, A., Hirani, S., Barnard, R., & Hilari, K. (2021). Solution Focused Brief Therapy in Post-Stroke Aphasia (SOFIA): Feasibility and acceptability results of a feasibility randomised wait-list controlled trial. *BMJ Open*, 11:e050308. doi: 10.1136/bmjopen-2021-050308

O'Hanlon, B. & Beadle, S. (1996). *A Field Guide to Possibility Land*. London, UK: Brief Therapy Press.

Ratner, H., George, E., & Iveson, C. (2012). *Solution Focused Brief Therapy: 100 Key Points and Techniques*. Hove, UK: Routledge.

Royal College of Speech and Language Therapists. (2005). *Clinical Guidelines*. Oxon: Speechmark Publishing.

Sekhon, J.K., Douglas, J., & Rose, M.L. (2015). Current Australian speech-language pathology practice in addressing psychological well-being in people with aphasia after stroke. *Speech Language Patholology*, 17(3), 252-262. doi:10.3109/17549507.2015.1024170

Simmons-Mackie, N. & Damico, J.S. (2011). Counseling and aphasia treatment: Missed opportunities. *Topics in Language Disorders*, 31(4), 336-351.

Smith, I.C. (2011). A qualitative investigation into the effects of brief training in solution-focused therapy in a social work team. *Psychology and Psychotherapy: Theory, Research and Practice*, 84(3), 335-348.

Stroke Association. (2015). Feeling overwhelmed. Accessed in https://www.stroke.org.uk/resources/feeling-overwhelmed.

Sung, J., Mayo, N., & Witting, A.B. (2018). A theoretical investigation of postmodern approaches used in medical settings: Solution-focused brief therapy. *The Family Journal*, 26(2), 200-207.

Thomas, S.A. & Lincoln, N.B. (2008). Predictors of emotional distress after stroke. *Stroke*, 39(4), 1240-1245. doi:10.1161/STROKEAHA.107.498279

Wichowicz, H.M., Puchalska, L., Rybak-Korneluk, A.M., Gąsecki, D., & Wiśniewska, A. (2017). Application of Solution-Focused Brief Therapy (SFBT) in individuals after stroke. *Brain Injury*, 31(11), 1507-1512.

Winkler, M., Bedford, V., Northcott, S., & Hilari, K. (2014). Aphasia blog talk: How does stroke and aphasia affect the carer and their relationship with the person with aphasia? *Aphasiology*, 28(11), 1301-1319. doi:10.1080/02687038.2014.928665

Zhang, A., Franklin, C., Currin-McCulloch, J., Park, S., & Kim, J. (2018). The effectiveness of strength-based, solution-focused brief therapy in medical settings: A systematic review and meta-analysis of randomized controlled trials. *Journal of Behavioral Medicine*, 41(2), 139-151.

4 Embracing technology with aphasia

Helen Kelly, Larry Masterson, Eileen O'Riordan
and Philip Scott

Technology, or more specifically Information and Communication Technology (ICT), relates to all technological methods used to manage information and aid communication technologies. It includes both computer and network hardware as well as their associated software. ICT is therefore a broad subject area which continues to advance and evolve at a fast pace, and so cannot be fully contained within the pages of this chapter. To harness the voice and perspectives of people living with aphasia, Helen (first author) explored with authors Larry, Eileen and Philip the impact that aphasia has on their use of technology in their daily lives. From the perspectives of the authors living with aphasia, *Health and Wellbeing* captures pertinent priorities around ICT for people with aphasia, more specifically, *Social Connection*, engaging in aphasia rehabilitation through *Telepractice*, and the accessibility of ICT for people with aphasia, i.e., *Digital Inclusion.* As one aim of this chapter is to educate speech and language therapy (SLT) students, 30 SLT students at University College Cork identified topics they would like to learn about in relation to technology and aphasia. Interestingly, many of their topic areas mirrored the priorities of our authors. First, we will provide a brief overview of ICT and how it may be used to enhance communication for people with aphasia. We will then explore ICT in relation to Social Connection, Telepractice, and Digital Inclusion.

Information and Communication Technology (ICT) and aphasia

ICT has become embedded in and permeates everyday society with 4.66 billion (59.5% of the global population) active Internet users worldwide and 79% of EU individuals using the Internet daily (Johnson, 2021). Although there is an upward trend in older adults, younger adults are more likely to use the Internet (Ofcom, 2020). Mobile technology devices are commonplace, with Smartphones currently being the most popular device for accessing the Internet (Ofcom, 2020). ICT has the potential to enhance quality of life, with the Internet making information more accessible (e.g., government and healthcare information) and everyday chores more efficient (e.g., online shopping and banking). Importantly, ICT can facilitate social connection, for example embracing the power of social media, providing a platform for people with aphasia to communicate with, advocate for, and support others living with aphasia. We will explore this further in this chapter. Technology can also be used to support or replace ways of communication, such as Alternative and Augmentative Communication (AAC). This is outside the scope of this chapter but we refer readers to Wallace (2020) for current evidence-based information related to AAC and aphasia. Authors with aphasia also use a range of assistive software, though not specifically designed for people with aphasia, to help them navigate post-stroke reading, writing and memory difficulties. See Caute and Woolf (2016), Caute et al. (2016), Cistola, Farrus, & van der Meulen (2021); Hux, Wallace, Brown, & Knollman-Porter (2021), and Szabo and Dittleman (2014) for examples of assistive software and how it may be employed by people with aphasia.

While sincerely hoping you are reading this chapter with the Covid-19 global pandemic firmly in your rear-view mirror, it must be noted that the impact of the pandemic has rapidly and substantially increased the utilization of technology in delivering healthcare and communications through necessity more than at any other time in history. This is changing the landscape of healthcare both now and potentially for the future. Continued advances in technology provide alternative ways of accessing healthcare information, consulting with healthcare professionals and accessing rehabilitation remotely. This synchronous aphasia rehabilitation will be explored further in this chapter, specifically Telepractice.

While this chapter focuses on synchronous ICT, it is important to note that a continuous plethora of computer-based therapy programs and applications are emerging that increase access to asynchronous aphasia rehabilitation. The availability of such programs can potentially intensify the rehabilitation of aphasia which is generally considered to improve therapy outcomes on a number of communication measures (Boghal, Teasell, & Speechley, 2003; Brady, Kelly, Godwin, Enderby, & Campbell, 2016; Cherney, Patterson, Raymer, Frymark, & Schooling, 2008; Patterson, Raymer & Cherney, 2020; Robey,

1998). The need for further high-quality research with larger sample sizes in computer-delivered aphasia rehabilitation has been noted but there is some evidence to suggest that computer-delivered aphasia rehabilitation is effective in comparison with no rehabilitation, and may be as effective as clinician-delivered therapy for some people with aphasia (Brady et al., 2016; Zheng, Lynch, & Taylor, 2016). Asynchronous ICT-delivered aphasia interventions have received generally positive feedback from people with aphasia and although some variation in personal perspectives and experiences exist, it is a generally satisfactory manner of rehabilitation for people with aphasia (Kearns, Kelly & Pitt, 2019). Co-author Larry highlighted the importance of Speech and Language Therapists' involvement in recommending appropriate software that is suitable for people with aphasia and the opportunity to trial aphasia rehabilitation Apps before purchasing.

The potential benefits of ICT that could be harnessed by people with aphasia seem limitless. However, to access the benefits of technology, one needs firstly to be able to acquire the relevant technological devices, understand complex set-up instructions and access mechanisms for reporting technological difficulties should they arise (Menger, Morris, & Salis, 2020). Secondly, our authors highlighted the essential need to access facilities such as strong, reliable broadband to facilitate Internet access, which is particularly poor in rural areas where people with aphasia are more isolated. Thirdly, the use of technology requires the user to have the technological, language and cognitive skills to be able to use the devices and to navigate the different software applications to fully capture ICT benefits. Herein lies the challenge for many people with aphasia and where the digital divide is most notable, yet where technology could potentially prove most beneficial. This is an area of concern that was highlighted as important to include in this chapter by the authors with aphasia.

Connecting with the person behind the screen

The World Happiness Report (Helliwell, Layard, Sachs, & De Neve, 2021) informs that social connection is vital for wellbeing and the prolonged experience of social distancing and increased isolation from people results in an increase of one's sense of loneliness. Social relationships are important for transactional exchanges but also for purely enjoyable interactions, "trading life stories and humorous anecdotes and engaging in playful, spontaneous exchanges" (Davidson, Howe, Worrall, Hickson, & Togher, 2008, p.337). Sadly, isolation is the daily lived experience of many people living with post-stroke aphasia due to physical and communication impairments, in addition to societal attitudinal and environmental barriers (Cruice, Worrall, & Hickson, 2006; Howe, Worrall, & Hickson, 2008; Parr, 2007; Simmons-Mackie, 2000). There is a resounding lack of awareness about aphasia globally (McCann, Tunnicliffe, & Anderson, 2013; McMenamin, Faherty, Larkin, & Loftus, 2020; Simmons-Mackie, Code, Armstrong, Stiegler, & Elman, 2002; Simmons-Mackie et al., 2020). This results in a communication-laden society largely inaccessible for people with aphasia, resulting in barriers to carrying out everyday activities independently as well as being involved in ordinary everyday communicative interactions. Indeed, people with aphasia are "marginalised by a communicatively inaccessible society" (Worrall, Rose, Howe, McKenna, & Hickson, 2007, p.135). The social network size and circle of friends often decreases for people living with aphasia (Code, 2003; Cruice et al., 2006; Davidson et al., 2008; Hilari & Northcott, 2006; Vickers, 2010) and often results in reductions in diversity, frequency and quality of interactions with both friends and acquaintances (Lee, Lee, Choi, & Pyun, 2015; Dalemans, De Witte, Wade, & van den Heuvel, 2010; Vickers, 2010) with some people with aphasia having no friends (Hilari & Northcott, 2006). The impact on people's lives is reflected in the fact that people with post-stroke aphasia experience significantly worse quality of life than people post-stroke without aphasia, particularly in relation to social relationships (Hilari, Needle, & Harrison, 2012). The frequency of depression is also higher for people with post-stroke aphasia (Hilari et al., 2012; Kauhanen et al., 2000; Hackett & Pickles, 2014; Hackett, Yapa, Parag, & Anderson, 2005). Lee et al. (2015) found that people with aphasia's experience of socially interacting with unfamiliar people was stressful. They report that reduced community integration was closely related to language abilities and lowered community integration had a negative effect on quality of life.

Retaining and establishing social networks and simply interacting with friends in conversation is one way of being connected to society (Grohn, Worrall, Simmons-Mackie, & Hudson, 2014; Moss et al., 2021; Northcott, Marshall, & Hilari, 2016). Being able to live a fruitful life with aphasia includes the ability to socially connect with other people living with aphasia for the purpose of social interaction as well as peer support (Brown, Worrall, Davidson, & Howe, 2010; Fotiadou, Northcott, Chatzidaki, & Hilari, 2014; Worrall et al., 2011). People with aphasia often want to share their experience of living with aphasia with their peers (Buhr, Hoepner, Miller, & Johnson, 2017; Fotiadou et al., 2014). Furthermore, preliminary evidence has shown one benefit of peer-befriending relates to a reduction in depression for people with post-stroke aphasia (Hilari et al., 2021). Technology can offer the opportunity to develop these social networks in addition to empowering, supporting and giving a voice to people living with aphasia. Social media exchange technologies can provide beneficial opportunities for peer-to-peer interactions (Moorhead et al., 2013). Social media can be used to provide peer, social and emotional support in relation to health communication (Buhr et al., 2017; Moorhead et al., 2013) and can foster encouragement, motivation and comfort in relation to living with aphasia (Buhr et al., 2017). There is a range of universally available social networking platforms for interactions with people with and without aphasia, for example Twitter, Facebook, Snapchat and Instagram. The most popular social networks worldwide are Facebook, followed by YouTube, WhatsApp, Facebook Messenger and Instagram (Statista, 2021).

Our authors living with aphasia have employed social media sites such as Facebook, Twitter and Instagram to extend their social networks, practise communication skills, raise awareness about aphasia, and support and advocate for people with aphasia. Larry established '*Different Strokes for Different Folks*', an online support group for people with aphasia in his local area on Facebook (Masterson, Sweeney, & O'Donnell, 2016) and Twitter (Masterson, 2018) and Philip created a Facebook Blog '*My Journey with Aphasia*' (Scott, 2019). Eileen and Philip attend UCC's online Aphasia Home Café where people with aphasia from all over Ireland, UK and further afield meet fortnightly to discuss a range of topics, supported by SLT students (Kelly & CTSoc, 2019). This opportunity for people with aphasia to meet outside of a traditional therapeutic environment has resulted in some exciting advocacy activities. For example, the café patrons with aphasia decided to use social media platforms for greater reach and influence during Aphasia Awareness month in 2021. Aphasia Home Café patrons also co-created a videoclip for an online event highlighting awareness about aphasia as well as the aphasia café (Kelly et al., 2020). Increasingly, people with post-stroke aphasia are discovering social media platforms as a way to connect with and support other people with aphasia from around the globe. Followed by thousands of social media followers, they share personal journeys and other information to spread awareness about aphasia, empowering them and giving them a voice to self-advocate. Beyond aphasia itself, people with aphasia are developing and expressing their creative side using technology, such as participating in online aphasia book clubs (for example, @*aphasiabookclub*), artistic expression, such as writing poetry (Neate, Roper, Wilson, & Marshall, 2019), creating comic strips (Tamburro, Neate, Roper, & Wilson, 2020), digital art (Neate, Roper, &

Wilson, 2020a) and creation of multimedia content (Neate, Roper, Wilson, Marshall, & Cruice, 2020b). Physical distance does not need to mean socially distant with ICT facilitating geographically diverse national and international networks for social connections, learning new pastimes and self-advocacy, much of which would not be possible without technology.

Aphasia and telepractice

Telemedicine technology can be used to (i) monitor the health of patients remotely; (ii) collect and transmit clinical data for later analysis, for example asynchronous rehabilitation, and (iii) interactive telemedicine which facilitates synchronous (real-time) communication between clinicians and patients (Flodgren, Rachas, Farmer, Inzitari, & Shepperd, 2015). Our discussions will focus on synchronous telemedicine, i.e., telepractice.

An unprecedented shift in healthcare provision

ASHA (2019) defines telepractice as "the application of telecommunications technology to the delivery of speech language pathology ... services at a distance by linking clinician to client ... for assessment, intervention and/or consultation". Interest in telepractice as a major service delivery model has amplified in response to the sudden outbreak of the coronavirus (Covid-19) global pandemic. The now protracted requirements for physical distancing in an effort to curb the spread of the disease has resulted in what Robbins et al. (2020, p.1) term as a global "unprecedented challenge for healthcare systems" which continually need to adapt to the ever-changing terrain. To protect people most vulnerable to contracting the disease, reducing patient contact in adherence to public health social distancing recommendations, and generally to reduce disease transmission, face-to-face medical visits were curtailed (Moradi, Babaee, Esfandiari, Lim, & Kordi, 2021; Robbins et al., 2020). Restrictions on public transportation systems (Moradi et al., 2021) and requirements for geographical travel permissions reduced convenient transport for hospital visit attendance. There were also public health concerns that people weren't seeking medical attention despite the medical need due to fears around contracting the disease. In addition, there was a need to protect the healthcare workforce from contracting Covid-19 by reducing patient contacts. Furthermore, many healthcare workers, including Speech and Language Therapists, were redeployed to serve the greatest medical need at Covid-19 testing centres and to contact tracing, reducing staff availability. This 'perfect storm' resulted in many rehabilitation services being suspended with healthcare facilities being restricted to the most urgent medical needs (Moradi et al., 2021). In response, many medical health appointments moved predominantly online, utilizing technology such as video calls for consultations (Moradi et al., 2021; Robbins et al., 2020).

Feasibility and effectiveness of telepractice in aphasia

Moradi et al. (2021) highlight the need for intense rehabilitation programmes being essential for the recovery of post-stroke patients and notes the risk of not providing early, intensive rehabilitation potentially causing a loss in recovery during the optimal recovery window. Although potentially not suitable for everyone, aphasia is one condition where high intensity and high dose interventions are considered to enhance patient recovery (Boghal et al., 2003; Brady et al., 2016; Cherney et al., 2008; Patterson et al., 2020; Robey, 1998) with telerehabilitation being one method of delivery. Pitt, Theodoros, Hill and Russell (2019, p.28) recognize remote speech and language therapy as being a "unique clinical setting where the interactions, resources and needs of consumers and clinicians differs from face-to-face". This is acknowledged by SLT professional bodies where the use of telepractice is approved when (i) it is based on current evidence-based practice, (ii) it is at least equivalent to standard clinical care, (iii) clinicians are appropriately familiar with the technology, (iv) the appropriacy of teletherapy is determined for each individual client, and (v) where there are gaps in evidence, policy or precedent, clinicians should employ the same decision-making process for other SLT interventions that do not yet have published evidence (ASHA, 2019; IASLT, 2020; RCSLT, 2020; SPA, 2020).

All authors with aphasia have had the opportunity to successfully engage in telepractice for their healthcare needs, which included SLT consultations, rehabilitation, and student paired communication skills practice in UCC's Communication Partner Programme. However, is telepractice as effective as face-to-face and is it an acceptable method of therapy from the perspective of the person with aphasia and their speech and language therapy clinicians?

Hall, Boisvert and Steele (2013) highlight that the first documented use of SLT telepractice and aphasia was in the 1970s (see Vaughn, 1976a, 1976b, 1977, 1981). Technology and rehabilitation methods have advanced since that time and literature supporting the use of telepractice is emerging. Hall et al. (2013) carried out a systematic review that included 10 studies: 60% of 153 participants had aphasia. In the included studies, telepractice included consultations, assessment, stroke outcome questionnaires and targeting aphasia related communication. While reporting that telepractice is an effective way to deliver healthcare services to people with aphasia, Hall et al. (2013) highlight the paucity of research around its use with this population. More recently, Weidner and Lowman (2020) conducted a systematic review where people with aphasia participated in half of the 125 included studies. Aphasia rehabilitation techniques ranged from progressive cueing hierarchies to target word retrieval (Agostini et al., 2014; Woolf et al., 2016); script training (Rhodes & Isaki, 2018), Promoting Aphasics' Communication Effectiveness (Macoir, Sauvageau, Boissy, Tousignant, & Tousignant, 2017), Verb Network Strengthening Treatment (Furnas & Edmonds, 2014) and Semantic Mediation for phonologic alexia (Getz, Snider, Brennan, & Friedman, 2016). Group therapy using videoconferencing was also found to be feasible and beneficial (Pitt et al., 2018, 2019; Steele, Baird, McCall ,& Haynes, 2014; Walker, Price, & Watson, 2018). Some studies supplemented rehabilitation with videoconference check-ins which were reported to enhance therapy outcomes (Choi, Park, & Paik, 2016; Kurland, Liu, & Stokes, 2018; Steele et al., 2014). Overall, telepractice was considered to have positive outcomes and established the feasibility of telepractice delivery of speech and language assessment and treatment with some equivalency compared to face-to-face delivery of aphasia therapy reported. Since this review, two recent studies carried out aphasia focused teletherapy: online group therapy (Pitt et al., 2019) and an individual language-oriented community-based programme supported by SLT students (Jacobs, Briley, Fang, & Ellis, 2021). Both studies found improvements in aphasia outcome measures: Assessment for Living with Aphasia and Comprehensive Aphasia Test (with some subtests reaching significance) (Pitt et al., 2019) and the WAB-RAQ (Jacobs et al., 2021).

Although the feasibility and some benefits of telepractice for aphasia rehabilitation are reported, many of the studies have relatively low-to-moderate methodological strength (e.g., small sample sizes, lack of control groups and poor setting/environment description); therefore, larger and more methodologically robust trials are needed to demonstrate efficacy (Cacciante et al., 2021; Hall et al., 2013; Weidner & Lowman, 2020). Øra et al. (2020a) carried out a pilot randomized controlled trial of post-stroke aphasia rehabilitation. Sixty-two people with aphasia were randomly allocated to aphasia rehabilitation by videoconference (5 hours weekly for 4 consecutive weeks) with usual care, or usual care alone. Both group scores increased significantly on the Communication Effectiveness Index with no significant group differences and no significant between-group differences in naming or auditory comprehension at the end of the rehabilitation period or 4 months post-randomization. However, the telerehabilitation group achieved a statistically significant increase in repetition score and Verb and Sentence Test compared to the usual care group at 4 months follow-up. Øra et al. (2020a) state that augmented telerehabilitation may be a viable aphasia rehabilitation model and recommend a larger definitive trial to confirm results. Very recently, Cacciante et al. (2021) undertook a systematic review and meta-analysis comparing telerehabilitation with face-to-face intervention for people with aphasia. They report that while the evidence is not adequate to guide clinical practice their findings suggest comparable language gains from both treatments, including functional communication skills.

Bridging clinical gains and 'virtual' reality

Realistic social communication situations are inherently difficult to create in a clinical setting and one challenge encountered in aphasia rehabilitation is the generalization of communication gains from the clinic to everyday communication settings. However, advances in technology now provide the exciting utilization of virtual reality (VR); providing opportunities to practise communication in enriched, complex and dynamic, virtual social situations. VR technology enables users to interact with computer-generated simulations of three-dimensional environments that may differ depending on the level of immersion, which is "the extent to which the system presents a vivid virtual environment while shutting out physical reality" (Cummings & Bailenson, 2016, p.3). Non-immersive VR uses devices such as desktop display, smartphone or tablet to explore and interact with the contents of the environment whereas immersive VR uses head-mounted displays which allow people to experience the environment as if they were physically present (Bryant, Brunner, & Hemsley, 2020; Cummings & Bailenson, 2016). The use of VR technology in rehabilitation contexts has been employed in a wide range of stroke-related health fields, including post-stroke hemiparesis (Housman, Scott, & Reinkensmeyer, 2009; Shin, Park, & Jang, 2015); post-stroke ataxia (dos Santos et al., 2018), balance and gait (de Rooij, van de Port, & Meijer, 2016), and quality of life after stroke (Shin et al., 2015). While results are promising, Laver et al. (2017) noted that the quality of VR research in post-stroke studies was generally low or moderate and called for improved, methodologically robust trials with larger sample sizes.

The use of technology to create virtual spaces and environments facilitates and mimics real-life communication situations, giving people with aphasia potential opportunities to practise their communication in real-world situations, beyond the clinical environment. An example of this is EVA Park where people with aphasia can interact synchronously with the clinician and/or with other people with aphasia while practising their communication skills in a range of different environments, for example bar, disco, beach, which can prompt different conversations (Marshall et al., 2016, 2018; Marshall, Devane, Talbot, & Wilson, 2021). Whilst still in its infancy, evidence of positive communication outcomes in the use of VR in aphasia rehabilitation is emerging (Bryant et al., 2020; Cao et al., 2021; Grechuta et al., 2019; Maresca et al., 2019; Vaezipour, Aldridge, Koenig, Theodoros, & Russell, 2021). Cao et al.'s (2021) systematic review on the effects of VR in post-stroke aphasia demonstrated a borderline positive clinical effect on language severity when compared with conventional rehabilitation therapy. However, they did not find that functional communication skills transferred from the virtual environment to real-world communication interactions and highlighted the need for further research with larger sample sizes to reach more definitive conclusions. (See Hayre, Muller, & Schrerer, 2021, to further explore VR in health and rehabilitation.)

Acceptability and satisfaction with telepractice

Our authors with aphasia highlighted advantages of telepractice, including eliminating long journeys, saving time and cost of transportation. The literature reports benefit for people living in geographically remote areas (Cason & Cohen, 2014; Hall et al., 2013; Moradi et al., 2021) and those with mobility difficulties (Cason & Cohen, 2014). Teletherapy reduces travel time and scheduling conflicts, and facilitates the maximization of resources (Hall et al., 2013; Pitt et al., 2018). It can give insight into people in their natural environments which is rarely achievable in face-to-face clinics (Cason & Cohen, 2014). The acceptability of telepractice by people living with aphasia and the facilitating clinicians is essential to its success and is explored below.

The perspectives of people with aphasia

Several recent studies explored satisfaction of telepractice rehabilitation with people with aphasia. Øra et al. (2020b) explored the acceptability of augmented telerehabilitation delivered to 30 people over two years which they measured through adherence and satisfaction with therapy. Protocol adherence was high with participants experiencing low and tolerable levels of technical faults (mainly internet connection causing delayed or interrupted sessions). Overall satisfaction with Telepractice was rated good/very good by 29/30 participants. Jacobs et al. (2021) found a high level of satisfaction with a 12-week telepractice rehabilitation programme with 22 people with aphasia who lived in geographically rural areas. Interestingly, satisfaction was highly predictive of effectiveness with a one-point increase in satisfaction associated with almost a 2-point increase in WAB-RAQ (Jacobs et al., 2021). Condon et al. (unpublished) evaluated satisfaction with telepractice from people at the early stage of their post-stroke journey. The Early Supported Discharge (ESD) team delivered physiotherapy, SLT and OT telerehabilitation to 27 people, eight of whom had aphasia. ESD telerehabilitation was found to be acceptable irrespective of age. Additionally, attendance and participant satisfaction over a 12-week TeleGAIN treatment block was high for all four participants in Pitt et al.'s (2019) study.

While people with aphasia were satisfied overall with aphasia rehabilitation through teletherapy, Øra et al. (2020b) recommend that technical expertise be provided to support this mode of rehabilitation. Technological equipment and software were installed for participants in Pitt et al.'s (2019) study and were provided with aphasia-accessible training and materials. Although they encountered unreliable video and audio connections during sessions, this was easily resolved. Students provided technical support in Jacobs et al.'s (2021) study, helping to set up the technical equipment and assisting participants. Condon et al. (unpublished) report that their participants ≥70 years of age rated significantly lower to the 'ease of use' domain of the usability questionnaire and over 50% of participants needed technical support. SLTs noted that while people with aphasia need adjustment time for the online environment and need support troubleshooting technology breakdowns, the majority were independent with technology by programme completion (Pitt et al., 2018; Simic et al., 2016).

The perspective of Speech and Language Therapists

Offering telepractice as a method of service delivery is strongly influenced by the views of those who provide the service (Dunkley, Pattie, Wilson, & McAllister, 2010; Wade, Elliot, & Hiller, 2014), in this case Speech and Language Therapists. Therefore, it is essential that factors which influence the acceptance of ICT use by healthcare professionals are considered (Holden & Karsh, 2010) as this may impact whether telepractice is offered as a rehabilitation option.

Kearns and Kelly (2022) explored the views of 15 SLTs through focus groups to identify clinical decision-making factors in relation to ICT in aphasia rehabilitation. Identified advantages of ICT included the opportunity to increase rehabilitation intensity and self-management. SLTs surveyed by Hill and Miller (2012), some of whom worked with people with aphasia, perceived benefits of telepractice such as improved access to SLT services and reduced travel time resulting in greater time and cost efficiency. Simic et al. (2016) interviewed two SLTs who rated satisfaction with teletherapy as high, noting it to be convenient and beneficial for people with aphasia. Pitt et al. (2018) interviewed three SLTs following the provision of their 12-week aphasia group therapy, who had received training in the rehabilitation technique and ICT prior to facilitating the therapy. They reported enjoying the online forum and considered it a feasible, worthwhile method of providing aphasia rehabilitation. The SLTs in Pitt et al. (2018) reported being able to build rapport with the therapy group members and, similar to Simic et al. (2016), found it took some time to adjust the role of facilitating communication in addition to managing the group dynamics in the online environment. Øra et al. (2020b) also found overall satisfaction with telerehabilitation was rated good/very good by two of three SLTs. Vaezipour et al. (2021) explored clinician acceptance, barriers and enablers of immersive VR technology in communication rehabilitation with 15 SLTs. The SLTs completed a usability survey, Simulator Sickness Questionnaire (SSQ), and were interviewed following the VR interaction. Overall SLTs rated usability as 'average', with low motion sickness and were positive about the usefulness of immersive VR and its potential for communication rehabilitation, noting the potential of functional communication skills transfer into real-world contexts.

While SLTs generally expressed overall positive experiences, several concerns were raised in relation to ICT-delivered aphasia rehabilitation. SLTs considered the limited evidence base for ICT-delivered rehabilitation, access to technology devices, Internet access (Kearns and Kelly, 2018), and a lack of assessment/treatment resources for telepractice (Hill & Miller, 2012). The most commonly reported barrier related to technological difficulties, such as audio/video quality disruptions, and instability and intermittent reliability of telecommunication connections negatively impacting clinician-patient interactions (Hill & Miller, 2012; Kearns and Kelly, 2022; Pitt et al., 2018; Simic et al., 2016), rendering communication more difficult than face-to-face (Simic et al., 2016). Adjusting to telepractice was compared to learning any new clinical skill, requiring "extra time, experience and effort" and as technical skills improved so did their confidence (Pitt et al., 2018, p.1046). The need for technological support and/or training to keep pace with ICT knowledge and skills was highlighted by several studies (Hill & Miller, 2012; Kearns and Kelly, 2018; Pitt et al., 2018).

Overall, patient and clinician perspectives need to be considered when introducing telepractice. Benefits to both are clear, however, challenges to successful implementation have been raised which largely focus on the need for technological support for both parties. Future research is needed with larger studies to ascertain the issues of concern of a larger body of clinicians and people with aphasia so benefits can be captured for the future provision of synchronous telepractice. Despite the challenges, SLTs and patients appear open to the engagement of synchronous telepractice in the rehabilitation of aphasia.

Narrowing the 'digital divide' – A Sisyphean task?

Aphasia and the Internet

The benefits of technology for people with aphasia are clear, providing opportunities to reduce social isolation, facilitate self-advocacy and enhance the ability to self-manage daily living. It can also provide opportunities to manage healthcare, for example facilitate timely access to health information or access aphasia rehabilitation. In fact, being able to access and benefit from the Internet is now established as a universal human right (Menger et al., 2020; McLeod, 2018) and people without access are disadvantaged and potentially digitally as well as socially isolated (Elman, 2001; Kelly et al., 2016; Menger et al., 2015).

Technological skills following stroke

Despite using technology prior to their stroke, authors Larry and Philip needed to relearn how to use technological devices and navigate the Internet post-stroke. Face-to-face accessible computer courses with aphasia-accessible materials and instruction have successfully helped people with aphasia relearn how to use technology (Egan, Worrall, & Oxenham, 2004; Kelly et al., 2016; Roper, Lancashire, Byrne, & Cruice, 2017). More recently, a co-designed aphasia-accessible online guide, 'Getting Online for People with Aphasia', with supporting videos is readily available (Stroke Association, 2021).

Interestingly, a client's age was a factor discussed by SLTs in the introduction of ICT rehabilitation (Kearns et al., 2018). Reflective of the general population (Ofcom, 2020), Menger et al. (2020) found age to be a perceived barrier to ICT use. Although Condon et al. (under review) reported some difficulties in accessing teletherapy in participants ≥70 years, Brennan et al. (2004) found age not to be a significant effect on performance in teletherapy. Age was also not a barrier for people with aphasia learning/relearning to use ICT, with participants aged 40-82 in Kelly et al.'s (2016) study.

Universal design ≠ aphasia accessible

The language skills required to successfully access and navigate technology, such as understanding audio content, reading online information, and contributing to online fora such as social networking sites, are reduced in aphasia (Menger et al., 2020). Menger et al. (2020) found that Internet use ranged from people with (and without) aphasia being fully independent to having someone act as a proxy for them; this was also true for participants without aphasia. Website design and social media interface often proves to be a barrier for people with communication difficulties such as aphasia (Egan et al., 2004; Elman, 2001; Kelly, et al., 2016; Menger et al., 2020; Roper, Grellmann, Neate, Marshall, & Wilson, 2018b). Elman (2001, p.897) poses the question 'What does an accessible website look like for someone who has moderate or severe aphasia?' and responds that the answer is not straightforward. The complexity of the layout of many websites, the number of steps required to complete an action (Cistola et al., 2021), and the inclusion of advertisements which produce additional visual and audio distractors, potentially compromises successful access and navigation by people with aphasia (Buhr et al., 2017). Our authors highlighted additional difficulties potentially interfering with concentration on technology-related tasks, such as post-stroke fatigue and brain fog which are experienced by many people post-stroke (Acciarresi, Bogousslavsky, & Paciaroni, 2014; Hinkle et al., 2017; Lerdal et al., 2009; McGeough et al., 2009). Co-comitant cognitive difficulties, such as working memory or executive functioning deficits, can further impact reading information, task monitoring, planning and organizing actions (Cistola et al., 2021). While some accessibility options are available on most technological devices, post-stroke hemiplegia difficulties can make them difficult to activate (Szabo & Dittelman, 2014). In addition, while online security is important, the oftentimes numerous security checks steps can be an additional barrier to access websites (Kelly et al., 2016; Buhr et al., 2017).

Singh (2000) outlines challenges of digital interfaces for people with lexical retrieval and reading impairment which result in difficulties formulating accurate search queries, navigational problems and understanding the retrieved information. Furthermore, the length and complexity of sentences used on websites is often a barrier for people with aphasia. Azios, Bellon-Harn, Dockens and Manchaiah (2019) note the readability of information on websites are generally at a too high level, with higher reading ability needed for aphasia rehabilitation websites compared to commercial or government websites. Ghidella, Murray, Smart, McKenna and Worrall (2005) evaluated the accessibility, readability and quality of five websites by people with aphasia and found that even websites considered to be 'accessible' are not necessarily high quality, and vice versa. Research on technologies designed specifically for people with post-stroke reading impairments is lacking (Cistola et al., 2021). Although technology is generally fast-paced, issues raised by Ghidella et al. (2005) are still prevalent 14 years later in Azios et al.'s 2019 study. For online information to be accessible to people with aphasia the involvement of people with aphasia is paramount (Worrall et al., 2007). Therefore, collaborative research needs to be undertaken at the design stages to ascertain the best reading levels for people with aphasia, and explore assistive technology effectiveness, such as voice recognition and text-to-speech software, in making online information more accessible to people with aphasia.

Social media sites designed to provide opportunities to socially connect can also be inaccessible for people with aphasia. Limited research has been undertaken related to the accessibility of social networking sites for people with aphasia. Roper et al. (2018b) undertook usability testing of four social networking sites (Facebook, Twitter, Tumblr and Pinterest) with four people with aphasia. Usability testing and interviews identified barriers and facilitators experienced by participants across social media sites. People reported more barriers for sites where they had little/no experience. Barriers included novel icons without supporting text, multiple steps to find action buttons, onscreen distractions, cognitive difficulties and, pertinent to aphasia, difficulties typing words. Participants with aphasia reported that facilitators included: previous experience with the platform, features such as predictive search, limited number of steps, and finding 'work-around' ways of navigating the system, for example typing their own name into the search bar to find their social media profile. A commonly reported factor of success was the support of a SLT or family members (Roper et al., 2018b). Burh et al. (2017) designed an aphasia-accessible social networking application (AphasiaWeb) for people with aphasia employing aphasia-accessible modifications to increase access and participation. People with aphasia trialled the software and provided feedback. They found that posts that were pictorial with captions and had low linguistic content were more highly engaged by participants. Feedback suggested that this was their preferred way of initiating conversations (Burh et al., 2017) which is similar to findings in other literature where photography provided people with aphasia a way of expressing concepts which, as a result of aphasia, were difficult to explain verbally (Brown et al., 2010; Miller & Happell, 2006). Baeir, Hoepner and Sather (2018) highlight that although most technologies and social networking applications are created to be universally accessed, there still remains a digital divide, with many people with aphasia only successfully navigating with personal support (Hoepner, Baier, Sather, & Clark, 2017; Kelly et al., 2016). They suggest that a universal social exchange platform needs to have aphasia-accessible functions such as "an uncomplicated interface, text-to-speech and speech-to-text functions, drawing and photograph/video capabilities" (Baeir et al., 2018, p.1339).

The bespoke nature of the training and the constant advancement of technology challenges inadequately available resources. It is not the sole responsibility of people with aphasia to learn/relearn engagement with technology. Galliers et al. (2012) found that people with aphasia did not always agree with SLTs in what makes an aphasia-accessible website. Technology companies have a responsibility to collaborate with their intended users as co-designers in a supported, authentic and meaningful way to ensure accessibility for everyone. Some small studies have demonstrated successful and authentic co-design with people with aphasia in informing the content, structure and format of websites (Kelly et al., 2018; Kerr, Hilari, & Litosseliti, 2010). For example, authors Helen and Philip collaborated with Computer Sciences, people with aphasia and SLTs to design a website for people with aphasia (Kelly et al., 2018). Indeed all technology-based programmes for people with aphasia should include them in the codesign process (for example, Galliers et al., 2012; 2017; Kearns et al., 2019; Neate et al., 2019, 2020a, 2020b; Roper, Davey, Wilson, Neate, & Grellmann, 2018a; Tamburro et al., 2020; Wilson et al., 2015).

Conclusion

This book chapter was written with authors from four different geographical locations and could not have been undertaken without technology. We provided an overview of benefits of technology which can enhance the lives of people living with aphasia, for example social connection and access to healthcare. Some of the challenges to equitable access to technology have been highlighted, and while there is no easy solution we suggest that people with aphasia are included as core members of the design and implementation of technology in order to narrow that 'digital divide'. As support is widely reported as aiding accessibility, there is a need for ongoing access to technology support for troubleshooting (Baier et al., 2018, Elman, 2001: Kelly et al., 2016; Roper et al., 2018a). Therefore, written and verbal technical support should be aphasia-accessible, supported by technical assistants trained to assist people with aphasia with their technical queries. Further research is needed to evaluate telepractice efficacy and to ascertain the perceptions of people with aphasia and the facilitating SLT clinicians. Several different outcome measures have been used to measure the feasibility, usability, acceptance, and satisfaction of telepractice. Establishing a core set of measures would facilitate comparison across studies. Optimum ways of making meaningful online social connections, empowering self-advocacy and giving a voice on social media platforms should be explored with people with aphasia. We need to turn technology development and design on its head. Rather than developing devices and software and then observing how people with aphasia can use it, there is an overwhelming need for Speech and Language Therapists, Human Computer Interaction specialists and people with aphasia to collaborate at the outset in order to make technology more accessible for all. Only then will we see a narrowing of the 'digital divide' for people with aphasia.

References

Acciarresi, M., Bogousslavsky, J., & Paciaroni, M. (2014). Poststroke fatigue: Epidemiology, clinical characteristics and treatment. *European Neurology*, 72, 255–261.

Agostini, M., Garzon, M., Benavides-Varela, S., De Pellegrin, S., Bencini, G., Rosadoni, S., Mancuso, M., Turolla, A., Meneghello, F., & Tonin, P. (2014). Telerehabilitation in poststroke anomia. *BioMed Research International*, 6. https://doi.org/10.1155/2014/706909

American Speech-Language-Hearing Association (ASHA). (2019). Telepractice: Overview. https://www.asha.org/Practice-Portal/ Professional-Issues/Telepractice/

Azios, J.H., Bellon-Harn, M., Dockens, A.L., & Manchaiah, V. (2019). Quality and readability of English-language internet information for aphasia. *International Journal of Speech-Language Pathology*, 21(1), 1–9. https://doi.org/10.1080/17549507.2017.1362034

Baier, C., Hoepner, J.K., & Sather, T.W. (2018). Exploring Snapchat as a dynamic capture tool for social networking in persons with aphasia. *Aphasiology*, 32(11), 1336–1359. https://doi.org/10.1080/02687038.2017.1409870

Bhogal, S., Teasell, R., & Speechley, M. (2003). Intensity of aphasia therapy, impact on recovery. *Stroke*, 34(4), 987–993.

Brady, M.C., Kelly, H., Godwin, J., Enderby, P., & Campbell, P. (2016). Speech and language therapy for aphasia following stroke. *Cochrane Database of Systematic Reviews*, 6. https://doi.org/10.1002/14651858.CD000425.pub4.

Brennan, D., Georgeadis, A., Baron, C., & Barker, L. (2004). The effect of videoconference-based telerehabilitation on story retelling performance by brain-injured subjects and its implications for remote speech-language therapy. *Telemedicine Journal and E-Health*, 10(2), 147–154. https://doi.org/10.1089/tmj.2004.10.147

Brown, K., Worrall, L., Davidson, B., & Howe, T. (2010). Snapshots of success: An insider perspective on living successfully with aphasia. *Aphasiology*, 24(10), 1267–1295. https://doi.org/10.1080/02687031003755429

Bryant, L., Brunner, M., & Hemsley, B. (2020). Review of virtual reality technologies in the field of communication disability: Implications for practice and research. *Disability and Rehabilitation: Assistive Technology*, 15(4), 365–372. https://doi.org/10.1080/17483107.2018.1549276

Buhr, H.R., Hoepner, J.K., Miller, H., & Johnson, C. (2017). AphasiaWeb: Development and evaluation of an aphasia-friendly social networking application. *Aphasiology*, 31(9), 999–1020. https://doi.org/10.1080/02687038.2016.1232361

Cacciante, L., Kiper, P., Garzon, M., Baldan, F., Federico, S., Turolla, A., & Agostini, M. (2021). Telerehabilitation for people with aphasia: A systematic review. *Journal of Communication Disorders*, 92. https://doi.org/10.1016/j.jcomdis.2021.106111

Cao, Y., Huang, X., Zhang, B., Kranz, G.S., Zhang, D.Z., Li, X., & Chang, J. (2021). Effects of virtual reality in post-stroke aphasia: A systematic review and meta-analysis. *Neurological Sciences*. https://doi.org/10.1007/s10072-021-05202-5

Cason, J. & Cohn, E.R. (2014). Telepractice: An overview and best practices. *ASHA Wire*, 23(1), 4–17. https://doi.org/10.1044/aac23.1.4

Caute, A., Cruice, M., Friede, A., Galliers, J., Dickinson, T., Green, R., & Woolf, C. (2016). Rekindling the love of books – a pilot project exploring whether e-readers help people to read again after a stroke. *Aphasiology*, 30(2–3), 290–319. https://doi.org/10.1080/02687038.2015.1052729

Caute, A. & Woolf, C. (2016). Using voice recognition software to improve communicative writing and social participation in an individual with severe acquired dysgraphia: An experimental single-case therapy study. *Aphasiology*, 30(2–3), 245–268. https://doi.org/10.1080/02687038.2015.1041095

Cherney, L., Patterson, J., Raymer, A., Frymark, T., & Schooling, T. (2008). Evidence-based systematic review: Effects of intensity of treatment and constraint-induced language therapy for individuals with stroke-induced aphasia. *Journal of Speech, Language and Hearing Research*, 51(5), 1282–1299.

Choi, Y.-H., Park, H.K., & Paik, N. (2016). A telerehabilitation approach for chronic aphasia following stroke. *Telemedicine Journal and E-Health*, 22(5), 434–440. https://doi.org/10.1089/tmj.2015.0138

Cistola, G., Farrus, M., & van der Meulen, I. (2021). Aphasia and acquired reading impairments: What are the high-tech alternatives to compensate for reading deficits? *International Journal of Language and Communication Disorders*, 56(1), 161–173. https://doi.org/10.1111/1460-6984.12569

Code, C. (2003). The quantity of life for people with chronic aphasia. *Neuropsychological Rehabilitation*, 13(3), 379–390. https://doi.org/10.1080/09602010244000255

Condon, M., Barrett, A., O'Regan, L., Pope, L., Goulding, M., Healy, L., O'Caoimh, R., & Hartigan, I. (unpublished). Tele-rehabilitation: Redefining stroke early supported discharge during the COVID-19. *Irish Medical Journal*.

Cruice, M., Worrall, L., & Hickson, L. (2006). Quantifying aphasic people's social lives in the context of non-aphasic peers. *Aphasiology*, 20(12), 1210–1225. https://doi.org/10.1080/02687030600790136

Cummings, J.J. & Bailenson, J.N. (2016). How immersive is enough? A meta-analysis of the effect of immersive technology on user presence. *Media Psychology*, 19(2), 272–309. https://doi.org/10.1080/15213269.2015.1015740

Dalemans, R.J., De Witte, L., Wade, D., & van den Heuvel, W. (2010). Social participation through the eyes of people with aphasia. *International Journal of Language & Communication Disorders*, 45(5), 537–550. https://doi.org/10.3109/13682820903223633

Davidson, B., Howe, T., Worrall, L., Hickson, L., & Togher, L. (2008). Social participation for older people with aphasia: The impact of communication disability on friendships. *Topics in Stroke Rehabilitation*, 15(4), 325–340. https://doi.org/10.1310/tsr1504-325

de Rooij, I.J.M., van de Port, I.G.L., & Meijer, J.-W.G. (2016). Effect of virtual reality training on balance and gait ability in patients with stroke: Systematic review and meta-analysis. *Physical Therapy*, 96(12), 1905–1918.

dos Santos, M.B., de Oliveira, C.B., dos Santos, A., Pires, C.G., Dylewski, V., & Arida, R.M. (2018). A comparative study of conventional physiotherapy versus robot-assisted gait training associated to physiotherapy in individuals with ataxia after stroke. *Behavioural Neurology, 2018*. doi: 10.1155/2018/2892065

Dunkley, C., Pattie, L., Wilson, L., & McAllister, L. (2010). A comparison of rural speech-language pathologists' and residents' access to and attitudes towards the use of technology for speech-language pathology service delivery. *International Journal of Speech-Language Pathology*, 12(4), 333–343. https://doi.org/10.3109/17549500903456607

Egan, J., Worrall, L., & Oxenham, D. (2004). Accessible Internet training package helps people with aphasia cross the digital divide. *Aphasiology*, 18(3), 265–280. https://doi.org/10.1080/02687030344000562

Elman, R.J. (2001). The Internet and aphasia: Crossing the digital divide. *Aphasiology*, 15(10–11), 895–899.

Flodgren, G., Rachas, A., Farmer, A., Inzitari, M., & Shepperd, S. (2015). Interactive telemedicine: Effects on professional practice and health care outcomes. *Cochrane Database of Systematic Reviews*, 9. https://doi.org/10.1002/14651858.CD002098.pub2.

Fotiadou, D., Northcott, S., Chatzidaki, A., & Hilari, K. (2014). Aphasia blog talk: How does stroke and aphasia affect a person's social relationships? *Aphasiology*, 28(11), 1281–1300. https://doi.org/10.1080/02687038.2014.928664

Furnas, D. W., & Edmonds, L. A. (2014). The effect of computerised Verb Network Strengthening Treatment on lexical retrieval in aphasia. *Aphasiology, 28*(4), 401–420. https://doi.org/10.1080/02687038.2013.869304

Galliers, J.R., Wilson, S., Roper, A., Cocks, N., Marshall, J., & Pring, T. (2012, August 12). Words are not enough: Empowering people with aphasia in the design process. The 12th Participatory Design Conference, Roskilde, Denmark. https://doi.org/10.1145/2347635.2347643

Getz, H., Snider, S., Brennan, D., & Friedman, R. (2016). Successful remote delivery of a treatment for phonologic Alexia via Telerehab. *Neuropsychological Rehabilitation*, 26(4), 584–609. https://doi.org/10.1080/09602011.2015.1048254

Ghidella, C., Murray, S., Smart, M., McKenna, K., & Worrall, L. (2005). Aphasia websites: An examination of their quality and communicative accessibility. *Aphasiology*, 19(12), 1134–1146. https://doi.org/10.1080/02687030500337871

Grechuta, K., Ballester, B.R., Munne, R.E.M., Bernal, T.U., Hervás, B.M., Mohr, B., Pulvermüller, F., San Segundo, R., & Verschure, P. (2019). Augmented dyadic therapy boosts recovery of language function in patients with nonfluent aphasia: A randomized controlled trial. *Stroke*, 50, 1270–1274. https://doi.org/10.1161/STROKEAHA.118.023729

Grohn, B., Worrall, L., Simmons-Mackie, N., & Hudson, K. (2014). Living successfully with aphasia during the first year post-stroke: A longitudinal qualitative study. *Aphasiology*, 28(12), 1405–1425. https://doi.org/10.1080/02687038.2014.935118

Hackett, M. & Pickles, K. (2014). Part I: Frequency of depression after stroke: An updated systematic review and meta-analysis of observational studies. *International Journal of Stroke*, 9(8), 1017–1025. https://doi.org/10.1111/ijs.12357

Hackett, M., Yapa, C., Parag, V., & Anderson. (2005). Frequency of depression after stroke. A systematic review of observational studies. *Stroke*, 36, 1330–1340.

Hall, N., Boisvert, M., & Steele, R. (2013). Telepractice in the assessment and treatment of individuals with aphasia: A systematic review. *International Journal of Telerehabilitation*, 5(1), 27–37.

Hayre, C.M., Muller, D., & Scherer, M.J. (2021). *Virtual Reality in Health and Rehabilitation*. London: Taylor & Francis.

Helliwell, J.F., Layard, R., Sachs, J.D., & De Neve, J.-E. (2021). *World Happiness Report*. Sustainable Development Solutions Network. https://worldhappiness.report/ed/2021/

Hilari, K. (2011). The impact of stroke: Are people with aphasia different to those without? *Disability and Rehabilitation*, 33(3), 211–218. https://doi.org/10.3109/09638288.2010.508829

Hilari, K. & Northcott, C. (2006). Social support in people with chronic aphasia. *Aphasiology*, 20(1), 17–36. https://doi.org/10.1080/02687030500279982

Hilari, K., Behn, N., James, K., Northcott, S., Marshall, J., Thomas, S., Simpson, A., Moss, B., Flood, C., McVicker, S., & Goldsmith, K. (2021). Supporting wellbeing through peer-befriending (SUPERB) for people with aphasia: A feasibility randomised controlled trial. *Clinical Rehabilitation*, 35(8), 1151-1163. https://doi.org/10.1177/0269215521995671

Hilari, K., Needle, J.J., & Harrison, K.L. (2012). What are the important factors in health-related quality of life for people with aphasia? A systematic review. *Archives of Physical Medicine and Rehabilitation*, 93(1), S86–S95. https://doi.org/10.1016/j.apmr.2011.05.028

Hill, A.J. & Miller, L.E. (2012). A survey of the clinical use of telehealth in speech-language pathology across Australia. *Journal of Clinical Practice in Speech-Language Pathology*, 14(3), 110–117.

Hinkle, J.L., Becker, K.J., Kim, J.S., Choi-Kwon, S., Saban, K.L., McNair, N., & Mead, G.E. (2017). Poststroke fatigue: Emerging evidence and approaches to management. A scientific statement for healthcare professionals from the American Heart Association. *Stroke*, 48, e159–e170. https://doi.org/10.1161/STR.0000000000000132

Hoepner, J.K., Baier, C., Sather, T.W., & Clark, M.B. (2017). A pilot exploration of Snapchat as an aphasia friendly social exchange technology at an Aphasia Camp. *Clinical Archives of Communication Disorders*, 2(1), 30–42. https://doi.org/10.21849/cacd.2016.00087

Holden, R.J. & Karsh, B.-T. (2010). The Technology Acceptance Model: Its past and its future in health care. *Journal of Biomedical Informatics*, 43, 159–172. https://doi.org/10.1016/j.jbi.2009.07.002

Housman, S.J., Scott, K.M., & Reinkensmeyer, D.J. (2009). A randomized controlled trial of gravity-supported, computer-enhanced arm exercise for individuals with severe hemiparesis. *Neurorehabilitation and Neural Repair*, 23(5), 505–514.

Howe, T.J., Worrall, L.E., & Hickson, L.M. (2008). Interviews with people with aphasia: Environmental factors that influence their community participation. *Aphasiology*, 22(10), 1092–1120. https://doi.org/10.1080/02687030701640941

Hux, K., Wallace, S.E., Brown, J.A., & Knollman-Porter, K. (2021). Perceptions of people with aphasia about supporting reading with text-to-speech technology: A convergent mixed methods study. *Journal of Communication Disorders*, 91. doi: 10.1016/j.jcomdis.2021.106098

Irish Association of Speech and Language Therapists, (IASLT). (2020). *IASLT Statement on Telepractice*. Dublin: IASLT.

Jacobs, M., Briley, P.M., Fang, X., & Ellis, C. (2021). Telepractice treatment for aphasia: Association between clinical outcomes and client satisfaction. *Telemedicine Reports*, 2(1), 118–124. https://doi.org/10.1089/tmr.2020.0024

Johnson, J. (2021). Internet usage in Europe. Statista. https://www.statista.com/topics/3853/internet-usage-in-europe/

Kauhanen, M., Korpelainen, J., Hiltunen, P., Määttä, R., Mononen, H., Brusin, E., Sotaniemi, K., & Myllylä. (2000). Aphasia, depression, and nonverbal cognitive impairment in ischaemic stroke. *Cerebrovascular Disease*, 10, 455–461.

Kearns, Á., & Kelly, H. (2022) ICT usage in aphasia rehabilitation – beliefs, biases, and influencing factors from the perspectives of speech and language therapists, *Aphasiology*, DOI: 10.1080/02687038.2022.2030462

Kearns, Á., Kelly, H., & Pitt, I. (2019). Self-reported feedback in ICT-delivered aphasia rehabilitation: A literature review. *Disability and Rehabilitation*. https://doi.org/10.1080/09638288.2019.1655803

Kelly, H., Horgan, A., Bell, S., Fleming, A., O'Sullivan, M., O'Riordan, E., Scott., P., Layton, P. & O'Sullivan, J. (2020). *Aphasia Café* [YouTube]. https://www.youtube.com/watch?v=bGFZ6Yz7TgM

Kelly, H. (2021). *AphasiaHomeCafé* [Twitter]. Aphasia Home Café. https://twitter.com/ AphasiaHomeCafe

Kelly, H., & Clinical Therapies Society. (2019). *Aphasia Café* [Facebook]. Aphasia Café. https://www.facebook.com/AphasiaCafe/

Kelly, H., Kearns, A., Daly, A., Murphy, A., Bernard, D., Cotter, J., O'Sullivan, J., Scott, P., & Mehigan, T. (2018). *Aphasia and Me*. Aphasia and Me. https://aphasiaandme.ucc.ie/

Kelly, H., Kennedy, F., Britton, H., McGuire, G., & Law, J. (2016). Narrowing the "digital divide" – facilitating access to computer technology to enhance the lives of those with aphasia: A feasibility study. *Aphasiology*, 30(2–3), 133–163. https://doi.org/10.1080/0 2687038.2015.1077926

Kerr, J., Hilari, K., & Litosseliti, L. (2010). Information needs after stroke: What to include and how to structure it on a website. A qualitative study using focus groups and card sorting. *Aphasiology*, 24(10), 1170–1196.

Kurland, J., Liu, A., & Stokes, P. (2018). Effects of a Tablet-based home practice program with telepractice on treatment outcomes in chronic aaphasia. *Journal of Speech, Language, and Hearing Research*, 61, 1140–1156. https://doi.org/10.1044/2018_JSLHR-L-17-0277

Laver, K., Lange, B., George, S., Deutsch, J., Saposnik, G., & Crotty, M. (2017). Virtual reality for stroke rehabilitation. *Cochrane Database of Systematic Reviews*, 11. https:// doi.org/10.1002/14651858.CD008349.pub4

Lee, H., Lee, Y., Choi, H., & Pyun, S.-B. (2015). Community integration and quality of life in aphasia after stroke. *Yonsei Medical Journal*, 56(6), 1694–1702. https://doi.org/10.3349/ ymj.2015.56.6.1694

Lerdal, A., Bakken, L.N., Kouwenhoven, S.E., Pedersen, G., Kirkevold, M., Finset, A., & Kim, H.S. (2009). Poststroke fatigue: A review. *Journal of Pain and Symptom Management*, 38(6), 928–949. https://doi.org/10.1016/j.jpainsymman.2009.04.028

Macoir, J., Sauvageau, V., Boissy, P., Tousignant, M., & Tousignant, M. (2017). In-home synchronous telespeech therapy to improve functional communication in chronic poststroke aphasia: Results from a quasi-experimental study. *Telemedicine Journal and E-Health*, 23(8), 630–639. https://doi.org/10.1089/tmj.2016.0235

Maresca, G., Maggio, M.G., Latella, D., Cannavo, A., De Cola, M.C., Portaro, S., Stagnitti, M.C., Silvestri, G., Torrisi, M., Bramanti, A., De Luca, R., & Calabro, R.S. (2019). Toward improving poststroke aphasia: A pilot study on the growing use of telerehabilitation for the continuity of care. *Journal of Stroke and Cerebrovascular Diseases*, 28(10), 1–9.

Marshall, J., Booth, T., Devane, N., Galliers, J., Greenwood, H., Hilari, K., Talbot, R., Wilson, S., & Woolf, C. (2016). Evaluating the benefits of aphasia intervention delivered in virtual reality: Results of a quasi-randomised study. *PLoS ONE*, 11(8). https://doi.org/10.1371/ journal.pone.0160381

Marshall, J., Devane, N., Edmonds, L., Talbot, R., Wilson, S., Woolf, C., & Zwart, N. (2018). Delivering word retrieval therapies for people with aphasia in a virtual communication environment. *Aphasiology*, 32(9), 1054–1074. https://doi.org/10.1080/02687038.2018 .1488237

Marshall, J., Devane, N., Talbot, R., & Wilson, S. (2021). Applications of virtual reality in aphasia therapy. In C.M. Hayre, D.J. Muller & M.J. Scherer (Eds), *Virtual Reality in Health and Rehabilitation*, 1st ed. (pp.199–214). London: Taylor & Francis.

Masterson, L. (2018). Different Strokes for Different Folks [Twitter]. Different Strokes for Different Folks. @DLDStrokeSupGrp

Masterson, L., Sweeney, N., & O'Donnell, K. (2016). Different Strokes for Different Folks [Facebook]. Different Strokes for Different Folks. https://www.facebook.com/donegalstrokesupportgroup

McCann, C., Tunnicliffe, K., & Anderson, R. (2013). Public awareness of aphasia in New Zealand. *Aphasiology*, 27(5), 568–580. https://doi.org/10.1080/02687038.2012.740553

McGeough, E., Pollock, A., Smith, L., Dennis, M., Sharpe, M., Lewis, S., & Mead, G. (2009). Interventions for post-stroke fatigue. *Cochrane Database of Systematic Reviews*, 3. https://doi.org/10.1002/14651858.CD007030.pub2.

McLeod, S. (2018). Communication rights: Fundamental human rights for all. *International Journal of Speech-Language Pathology*, 20(1), 3–11.

McMenamin, R., Faherty, K., Larkin, M., & Loftus, L. (2020). An investigation of public awareness and knowledge of aphasia in the West of Ireland. *Aphasiology*. https://doi.org/10.1080/02687038.2020.1812047

Menger, F., Morris, J., & Salis, C. (2015). Aphasia in an Internet age: Wider perspectives on digital inclusion. *Aphasiology*, 30(2–3), 112–132. https://doi.org/10.1080/02687038.2015.1109050

Menger, F., Morris, J., & Salis, C. (2020). The impact of aphasia on Internet and technology use. *Disability and Rehabilitation*, 42(21), 2986–2996.

Moorhead, S.A., Hazlett, D.E., Harrison, L., Carroll, J.K., Irwin, A., & Hoving, C. (2013). A new dimension in health care: Systematic review of the uses, benefits, and limitations of social media for health communication. *Journal of Medical Internet Research*, 15(4), 85–112. https://doi.org/10.2196/jmir.1933

Moradi, V., Babaee, T., Esfandiari, E., Lim, S.B., & Kordi, R. (2021). Telework and telerehabilitation programs for workers with a stroke during the COVID-19 pandemic: A commentary. *IOS Press*, 77–80. https://doi.org/10.3233/WOR-203356

Moss, B., Northcott, S., Behn, N., Monnelly, K., Marshall, J., Thomas, S., Simpson, A., Goldsmith, K., McVicker, S., Flood, C., & Hilari, K. (2021). 'Emotion is of the essence … Number one priority': A nested qualitative study exploring psychosocial adjustment to stroke and aphasia. *International Journal of Language and Communication Disorders*. https://doi.org/10.1111/1460-6984.12616

Neate, T, Roper, A., Wilson, S., & Marshall, J. (2019). Empowering expression for users with aphasia through constrained creativity. *Proceedings of the 2019 CHI Conference on Human Factors in Computing Systems*. CHI '19, New York, USA. https://doi.org/10.1145/3290605.3300615

Neate, T., Roper, A., & Wilson, S. (2020). Painting a picture of accessible digital art. *Proceedings of the 22nd International ACM SIGACCESS Conference on Computers and Accessibility*. ASSETS '20, Athens, Greece. https://doi.org/10.1145/3373625.3418019

Neate, T., Roper, A., Wilson, S., Marshall, J., & Cruice, M. (2020). CreaTable content and tangible interaction in aphasia. *Proceedings of the 2020 CHI Conference on Human Factors in Computing Systems*, 1–14. https://doi.org/10.1145/3313831.3376490

Northcott, S., Marshall, J., & Hilari, K. (2016). What factors predict who will have a strong social network following a stroke? *Journal of Speech, Language, and Hearing Research*, 59(4), 772–783. https://doi.org/10.1044/2016_JSLHR-L-15-0201

Ofcom. (2020). *International Communications Market Report*. https://www.ofcom.org.uk/research-and-data/multi-sector-research/cmr/cmr-2020

Øra, H.P., Kirmess, M., Brady, M.C., Partee, I., Hognestad, R. ., Johannessen, B.B., Thommessen, B., & Becker, F. (2020a). The effect of augmented speech-language therapy delivered by telerehabilitation on poststroke aphasia: A pilot randomized controlled trial. *Clinical Rehabilitation*, 34(3), 369–381. https://doi.org/Frank

Øra, H.P., Kirmess, M., Brady, M.C., Sorli, H., & Becker, F. (2020b). Technical features, feasibility, and acceptability of augmented telerehabilitation in post-stroke aphasia: Experiences from a randomized controlled trial. *Frontiers in Neurology*, 11, 1–12.

Parr, S. (2007). Living with severe aphasia: Tracking social exclusion. *Aphasiology*, 21(1), 98–123. https://doi.org/10.1080/02687030600798337

Patterson, J., Raymer, A., & Cherney, L. (2020). Treatment intensity in aphasia rehabilitation. In P. Coppins & J. Patterson (Eds), *Aphasia Rehabilitation Clinical Challenges* (pp.291–329). Jones & Bartlett Learning.

Pitt, R., Hill, A.J., Theodoros, D., & Russell, T. (2018). "I definitely think it's a feasible and worthwhile option": Perspectives of speech-language pathologists providing online aphasia group therapy. *Aphasiology*, 32(9), 1031–1053. https://doi.org/10.1080/02687038.2018.1482403

Pitt, R., Theodoros, D., Hill, A.J., & Russell, T. (2019). The development and feasibility of an online aphasia group intervention and networking program – TeleGAIN. *International Journal of Speech-Language Pathology*, 21, 23–36. https://doi.org/10.1080/17549507.2017.1369567

Rhodes, N. & Isaki, E. (2018). Script training using telepractice with two adults with chronic non-fluent aphasia. *International Journal of Telerehabilitation*, 10(2), 89–103.

Robbins, T., Hudson, S., Ray, P., Sankar, S., Patel, K., Randeva, H., & Arvanitis, T. (2020). COVID-19: A new digital dawn? *Digital Health*, 6, 1–3. https://doi.org/10.1177/2055207620920083

Robey, R. (1998). A meta-analysis of clinical outcomes in the treatment of aphasia. *Journal of Speech, Language and Hearing Research*, 41(1), 172–187.

Roper, A., Davey, I., Wilson, S., Neate, T., Marshall, J., & Grellmann, B. (2018a). Usability testing – An aphasia perspective. *ASSETS '18 Proceedings of the 20th International ACM SIGACCESS Conference on Computers and Accessibility*, 102–106. https://doi.org/10.1145/3234695.3241481

Roper, A., Grellmann, B., Neate, T., Marshall, J., & Wilson, S. (2018b). Social networking sites: Barriers and facilitators to access for people with aphasia. *Aphasiology*, 32(Sup1), 176–177. https://doi.org/10.1080/02687038.2018.1486387

Roper, A., Lancashire, T., Byrne, R., & Cruice, M. (2017). Meaningful individualised goal-setting within a computer training course for adults with chronic aphasia. Poster presentation at the Nordic Aphasia Conference, 2017.

Royal College of Speech and Language Therapists (RCSLT). (2020). *Telehealth Guidance.* https://www.rcslt.org/members/delivering-quality-services/telehealth/telehealth-guidance/

Scott, P. (2019). My journey with Aphasia [Facebook]. *My Journey with Aphasia.* https://www.facebook.com/My-journey-with-aphasia-513067292761367

Shin, J.-H., Park, S.B., & Jang, S.H. (2015). Effects of game-based virtual reality on health-related quality of life in chronic stroke patients: A randomized, controlled study. *Computers in Biology and Medicine,* 63, 92–98. https://doi.org//10.1016/j.compbiomed.2015.03.011

Simic, T., Leonard, C., Laird, L., Cupit, J., Hobler, F., & Rochon, E. (2016). A usability study of Internet-based therapy for naming deficits in aaphasia. *Speech-Language Pathology,* 25(4), 642–653. https://doi.org/10.1044/2016_AJSLP-15-0030

Simmons-Mackie, N. (2000). Social approaches to management of aphasia. In L.E. Worrall & C.M. Frattali (Eds), *Neurogenic Communication Disorders: A Functional Approach* (pp.162–189). New York: Thieme.

Simmons-Mackie, N, Worrall, L., Shiggins, C., Isaksen, J., McMenamin, R., Rose, T., Guo, Y.E., & Wallace, S.J. (2020). Beyond the statistics: A research agenda in aphasia awareness. *Aphasiology,* 34(4), 458–471. https://doi.org/10.1080/02687038.2019.1702847

Simmons-Mackie, N., Code, C., Armstrong, E., Stiegler, L., & Elman, R. (2002). What is aphasia? Results of an international study. *Aphasiology,* 16(8), 837–848. https://doi.org/10.1080/02687030244000185

Singh, S. (2000). Designing intelligent interfaces for users with memory and language limitations. *Aphasiology,* 14(2), 157–177. https://doi.org/10.1080/026870300401531

Speech Pathology Australia (SPA). (2020). Telepractice. https://www.speechpathologyaustralia.org.au/SPAweb/Resources_for_Speech_Pathologists/Professional_Resources/HTML/Telepractice.aspx

Statista. (2021). Most popular social networks worldwide as of January 2021. https://www.statista.com/statistics/272014/global-social-networks-ranked-by-number-of-users/

Steele, R.D., Baird, A., McCall, D., & Haynes, H. (2014). Combining teletherapy and online language exercises in the treatment of chronic aphasia: An outcome study. *International Journal of Telerehabilitation,* 6(2), 3–20. https://doi.org/10.5195/ijt.2014.6157

Stroke Association. (2021). Getting online for people with aphasia. https://www.stroke.org.uk/what-is-aphasia/communication-tools/getting-online-people-aphasia

Szabo, G. & Dittelman, J. (2014). Using mobile technology with individuals with aphasia: Native iPad features and everyday apps. *Seminars in Speech and Language,* 35(5), 5–16. https://doi.org/10.1055/s-0033-1362993

Tamburro, C., Neate, T., Roper, A., & Wilson, S. (2020). Accessible creativity with a comic spin. The 22nd International ACM SIGACCESS Conference on Computers and Accessibility. https://doi.org/10.1145/3373625.3417012

Vaezipour, A., Aldridge, D., Koenig, S., Theodoros, D., & Russell, T. (2021). "It's really exciting to think where it could go": A mixed-method investigation of clinician acceptance, barriers and enablers of virtual reality technology in communication rehabilitation. *Disability and Rehabilitation*. https://doi.org/10.1080/09638288.2021.1895333

Vaughn, G. (1981). Efficacy of remote delivery of aphasia treatment by tel-communicology. Veterans Administrations Rehabilitation Research and Development Proposal.

Vaughn, G.R. (1976a). Innovative systems for improved and expanded delivery of health care and the exchange of medical information and medical information services for veterans with speech disorders. Final report, Tel- Communicology: VAMED #10. Veterans Administration Exchange of Medical Information Service.

Vaughn, G.R. (1976b). Tel-communicology: Health-care delivery system for persons with communicative disorders. *ASHA*, 18, 13–17.

Vaughn, G.R. (1977). Tel-communicology: Outreach services for rural Americans with communication disorders. Congressional Record-House; 11981-2.

Vickers, C.P. (2010). Social networks after the onset of aphasia: The impact of aphasia group attendance. *Aphasiology*, 24(6–8), 902–913. https://doi.org/:10.1080/02687030903438532

Wade, V., Elliot, J., & Hiller, J. (2014). Clinician acceptance is the key factor for sustainable telehealth services. *Qualitative Health Research*, 24(5), 682–694. https://doi.org/10.1177/1049732314528809

Walker, J.P., Price, K., & Watson, J. (2018). Promoting social connections in a synchronous telepractice, aphasia communication group. *Perspectives of the ASHA Special Interest Groups*, 3(18), 32–42.

Wallace, S. (2020). Complementing therapy using multimodal strategies. In P. Coppens & J. Patterson (Eds), *Aphasia Rehabilitation Clinical Challenges* (pp.249–290). Boston, MA: Jones & Bartlett Learning.

Weidner, K. & Lowman, J. (2020). Telepractice for adult Speech-Language-Pathology Services: A systematic review. *Perspectives of the ASHA Special 326 Interest Groups*, 5, 326–338.

Wilson, S., Roper, A., Marshall, J., Galliers, J.R., Devane, N., Booth, T., & Woolf, C. (2015). Codesign for people with aphasia through tangible design languages. *CoDesign*, 11(1), 21–34. https://doi.org/10.1080/15710882.2014.997744

Woolf, C., Caute, A., Haigh, Z., Galliers, J., Wilson, S., Kessie, A., Hirani, S., Hegarty, B., & Marshall, J. (2016). A comparison of remote therapy, face to face therapy and an attention control intervention for people with aphasia: A quasi-randomised controlled feasibility study. *Clinical Rehabilitation*, 30(4), 359–373.

Worrall, L., Sherratt, S., Rogers, P., Howe, T., Hersch, D., Ferguson, A., & Davidson, B. (2011). What people with aphasia want: Their goals according to the ICF. *Aphasiology*, 25(2), 309–322. https://doi.org/10.1080/02687038.2010.508530

Worrall, L., Rose, T., Howe, T., McKenna, K., & Hickson, L. (2007). Developing an evidence-base for accessibility for people with aphasia. *Aphasiology*, 21(1), 124–136. https://doi.org/10.1080/02687030600798352

Zheng, C., Lynch, L., & Taylor, N. (2016). Effect of computer therapy in aphasia: A systematic review. *Aphasiology*, 30(2–3), 211–244. https://doi.org/10.1080/02687038.2014.996521

5 Assessing mental capacity for people with aphasia

Mark Jayes

Introduction

In different parts of the world, the assessment of decision-making ability, or mental capacity, is an important and increasingly common aspect of clinical practice for speech and language therapists (SLTs) who work with adults. Our clinical training as SLTs means that we have unique strengths to bring to mental capacity assessment, in terms of our specialist understanding of how to identify and support the needs of people who have communication disorders such as aphasia. This group is particularly vulnerable during the mental capacity process and requires individualized communication support to maximize their participation in decision making. This chapter provides an overview of UK mental capacity legislation and outlines our roles and responsibilities as mental capacity assessors, communication facilitators, educators and trainers. It also suggests practical approaches to completing robust assessments for people with aphasia.

What is mental capacity?

Mental capacity, or decision-making capacity, refers to the ability to make a decision (OPSI, 2005). Being able to make decisions about different aspects of our lives, for example what we eat, which clothes we wear, where we live, how we spend our time and money, and which healthcare interventions we consent to undergo, enables us to exercise our personal autonomy and express who we are as individuals. As you are reading this, imagine how it might feel if you were not able to make these decisions, or were not given opportunities to make them.

Involving the people we work with in decisions about their care and treatment is fundamental to ethical practice. Most Western ethical frameworks used in healthcare promote respect for individual autonomy (Beauchamp & Childress, 2008; Seedhouse, 2009). We respect people's autonomy when we seek informed consent before we carry out any speech and language therapy intervention. Similarly, we respect individual autonomy when we involve the people we work with in decisions about their treatment and care. This helps us to make our practice 'patient-centred' (Elwyn et al., 2012).

Current UK government policy promotes the involvement of people in decisions about their care. One mechanism for achieving this is through the provision of accessible information about health conditions and treatment options (e.g., Accessible Information Standard, NHS England, 2015). Another is through mental capacity legislation. The next section provides an overview of this legislation and our legal obligations when working with people with aphasia and other communication disorders.

What does mental capacity legislation say?

Across the UK, different legal frameworks are designed to protect and promote people's decision-making rights. In England and Wales, the relevant legislation is the Mental Capacity Act (MCA; OPSI, 2005), whereas in Scotland it is the Adults with Incapacity (Scotland) Act (AISA; Scottish Government, 2000) and in Northern Ireland it is the Mental Capacity Act (Northern Ireland) (MCA NI; TSO, 2016). These different legal frameworks all describe when and how mental capacity should be assessed and have common principles. For the purposes of this chapter, we will focus on the legal framework provided by the Mental Capacity Act (2005) but identify aspects of the other frameworks that are relevant to SLTs working in Scotland and Northern Ireland. Each law has its own Code of Practice, which is like an operating manual that helps people understand and apply the law. The Code of Practice can be a useful starting point for those new to this area of practice, as it describes the law and our legal responsibilities in more accessible language than the statutes themselves. Each legal framework is based on a set of principles. These principles are incredibly useful as they summarize the most important aspects of the law and can serve as a helpful guide when we feel confused or lack confidence about implementing the law. In England and Wales, the MCA has five principles. These are shown in Figure 5.1. For an overview of the legal principles that apply in Scotland and Northern Ireland, see Bailey (2018).

Importantly, the first statutory principle tells us that we should assume anyone we work with has intact decision-making capacity, unless we can

A person must be assumed to have capacity unless it can be established he lacks capacity.

A person is not to be treated as unable to make a decision unless all practicable steps to help him do so have been taken without success.

A person is not to be treated as unable to make a decision merely because he makes an unwise decision.

An act done, or decision made, under this Act for or on behalf of a person who lacks capacity must be done, or made, in his best interests.

Before the act is done, or the decision made, regard must be had to whether the purpose for which it is needed can be effectively achieved in a way that is less restrictive of the person's rights and freedom of action.

Figure 5.1 The principles of the Mental Capacity Act 2005 (OPSI, 2005, paragraph 1(2)).

establish through a mental capacity assessment that the person lacks capacity. The second principle requires anyone involved in a person's care to provide decision-making support if this is needed. This support can be provided before or during a mental capacity assessment. For people living with communication disabilities caused by conditions such as aphasia, this support is likely to be in the form of the use of inclusive communication approaches to enable individuals to access information about decisions and demonstrate their decision-making abilities. Therefore, the second principle really helps to identify and promote the important role of speech and language therapists in mental capacity assessments and supported decision making. These first two principles are common to all UK legislation.

The third principle relates to unwise decisions. We all make what others might perceive to be unwise decisions from time to time and this is our right as autonomous beings. For example, some people choose to smoke and drink alcohol, which many people would argue are risky activities; other people might choose to travel without health insurance, which again some people might consider to be unwise. We use our own values, beliefs, and experiences to decide what we think is wise or unwise. The law says we need to respect a person's right to make what we think might be an unwise decision and we should not conclude that they lack capacity to make the decision. Despite the law stating this clearly, some professionals still make value-based judgements of the wisdom of people's choices and decisions during assessments of their capacity; this appears to be motivated in part by a need to protect the individual from harm (Murrell & McCalla, 2016). After all, the need to do no harm is a central tenet of most Western ethical frameworks that we use in healthcare. Similarly, mental capacity law states that we should not decide to complete a mental capacity assessment and we cannot make decisions about a person's mental capacity on the basis of their age, behaviour or simply because they have a particular diagnosis or disability. For example, it would be unlawful for a professional to conclude that a person lacked capacity because they had aphasia. Instead, the professional needs to complete a process of mental capacity assessment if they think the individual may have difficulty making a decision. In all UK legal frameworks, capacity is defined as time and decision-specific. This means that we need to complete a separate capacity assessment for each decision a person needs to make at the time they need to make it. The MCA Code of Practice explicitly states that a capacity assessment should not be used to make judgements about a person's general decision-making ability (DCA, 2007, paragraph 4.4).

All UK laws define a two-stage process of capacity assessment. The first stage requires assessors to establish if there is a potential cause for the difficulty the person has in making the decision. The MCA states that an individual may lack capacity if it can be determined that they have an impairment or disturbance of their mind or brain which may affect their ability to make decisions (MCA, paragraph 2(1)). Different health conditions might cause an impairment or disturbance; these include temporary disturbances caused by delirium or alcohol/drug effects and longer-term effects due to neurological change, mental health conditions or learning disability. Aphasia caused by stroke would constitute an impairment under this definition. If the person being assessed does not appear to have such an impairment or disturbance, we need to conclude that they have capacity to make the decision and discontinue the process of assessment.

If the person does have an impairment or disturbance, the second stage of capacity assessment should be carried out. This involves checking whether the person can make the decision, with whatever support they need (see principle two above). The different UK legal frameworks prescribe slightly different functional tests of decision making. These require the professional to examine the person's decision-making abilities in order to determine if the person has any difficulty. The functional tests for each UK legal framework are shown below in Table 5.1. If the professional finds evidence that the person has difficulty with one or more of these abilities, then they should conclude that the person lacks capacity to make that decision. It is important to note here that the law is clear it is the professional's responsibility to find evidence that a person lacks capacity, not the person's responsibility to demonstrate or prove that they can make the decision (remember principle one above).

Principles four and five of the MCA relate to what happens when a mental capacity assessment concludes that a person lacks mental capacity. In this situation, anyone concerned with the person's welfare (family members, friends, healthcare professionals, independent advocates) needs to make a decision about what should happen in the person's best interests. They should discuss the advantages and disadvantages of each decision option. It is essential that this discussion includes consideration of which option the person appears to prefer and any past or present wishes and preferences the person has expressed in relation to the decision. For example, even though a person may not have capacity to make the decision, they may have expressed clearly which option they prefer during the capacity assessment.

In addition, they may have discussed this type of decision with their family in the past and engaged in some formal or informal advance care planning activity. Advance care planning refers to statements and decisions made by people when they still have mental capacity about how they wish to be cared for and treated at a future time when they lack mental capacity. UK mental capacity legislation provides different mechanisms to enable people

Table 5.1 Comparison of functional tests of decision-making across UK legal frameworks.

Ability tested	MCA (2005)	AISA (2000)	MCA NI (2016)
Understanding of decision Information	Ability to understand **relevant** information related to the decision.		
Retention of decision information	Ability to retain information for as long as it takes to **make a decision**.	Ability to retain information long enough to make a decision **and act on it**.	Ability to retain for information as long as it takes to **make a decision**.
Consideration of decision information	Ability to **use or weigh** information in order to make a decision.	Ability to use or weigh **and act on** information.	Ability to use or weigh information **and appreciate its relevance**.
Communication of a decision	Ability to communicate a decision using **any means**.		

to engage in advance care planning. For example, an individual can make an 'advance statement' (in England and Wales), 'advance care plan' (in Northern Ireland) or 'anticipatory care plan' (in Scotland) specifying their wishes and preferences for future care and living arrangements. An individual can also make an 'advance decision' or 'advance directive' to refuse a specific type of treatment, including artificial nutrition and hydration. People can also make advance decisions to nominate others to make decisions on their behalf at a future time: this type of arrangement is called a 'power of attorney'. For more information about advanced care planning, see Volkmer (2016).

If it is possible to ascertain what the person would like to happen in relation to the specific question, this information should form an important part of the best interests decision-making process. It is also essential to consider the person's values and beliefs when considering what might be in their best interests. This is why it is vital to include people who know the person very well, and ideally the person themselves, in these discussions. For more information on best interests decision-making, see the MCA Code of Practice (2007) section 4.

This brief introduction to UK mental capacity legislation is not a substitute for training in, or for more in-depth reading about, mental capacity assessment. There are many sources of helpful information relating to mental capacity law and its practical application. Some examples are shown in Figure 5.2. As SLTs we do not need to be experts in this legislation but we do need to develop a degree of 'legal literacy' – we need to be able to apply legal principles to our ethical practice. It is important to note that the legislation in England and Wales and Scotland is currently being amended, whilst in Northern Ireland, the legislation has not yet been fully implemented. This underlines the need to remain regularly updated about our legal responsibilities through training or reading.

How does mental capacity relate to our work with people with aphasia?

There is a small but growing evidence base relating to mental capacity assessment for people with aphasia. For a summary of this, see Suleman and Hopper (2015) and for more recent work in the UK, see McCormick, Bose and Marinis (2017) and Borrett and Gould (2020). Most recent literature has focused on exploration of professionals' experiences of assessment and descriptions of their practice. There is a dearth of literature exploring the experiences of

- Check your employer's mental capacity law guidance and policies

- Speak to your organization's mental capacity lead or legal team

- Read the Code of Practice for the law for your jurisdiction

- Read good practice recommendations in the NICE Guideline NG108 'Decision-making and mental capacity' available at: https://www.nice.org.uk/guidance/ng108

- Review RCSLT's mental capacity guidance on their website: https://www.rcslt.org/speech-and-language-therapy/guidance-for-delivering-slt-services/supported-decision-making-and-mental-capacity

- Review accessible legal summaries, commentaries, webinars available at

   -Barrister Alex Ruck Keene's "Mental Capacity Law and Policy" website: https://www.mentalcapacitylawandpolicy.org.uk/

   -39 Essex Chambers legal practice website: https://www.39essex.com/resources-and-training/mental-capacity-law/

- Review practical guidance and resources on the Social Care Institute for Excellence website:

   -https://www.scie.org.uk/atoz/?f_az_subject_thesaurus_terms_s=mental+capacity&st=atoz

Figure 5.2 Sources of guidance on mental capacity law.

people with aphasia in relation to mental capacity assessment. The limited evidence we do have suggests that people with aphasia want to be supported to participate in decision making that directly affects them and do not want others to make decisions on their behalf (Kagan & Kimmelman, 1995).

People with aphasia may experience communication difficulties in the presence or absence of concomitant cognitive difficulties. The precise nature of the relationship between linguistic abilities and decision-making abilities is still debated. However, we know that it is possible for a person with aphasia's inherent decision-making abilities to remain intact despite their linguistic difficulties (Kim, Suleman, & Hopper, 2020). Despite this, other people, including healthcare professionals, may make inaccurate assumptions about the relationship between communication disability and mental capacity. There is evidence to suggest that some professionals may assume people lack mental capacity simply because they have a communication disability. In a survey of SLTs working with people in with aphasia in England, 71% respondents reported they believed that their multidisciplinary colleagues assumed that people with aphasia lacked capacity (McCormick et al., 2017).

The legal definition and, therefore, testing of decision-making capacity in many jurisdictions across the world involves the use of cognitive-linguistic abilities (Suleman & Hopper, 2015). As noted above, the legal tests for capacity in the UK involve the examination of a person's ability to understand, retain and use information in order to make a decision, which the person needs to communicate to the assessor(s). Performance on these tests is therefore predicated on the ability to communicate; the presence of a communication disorder may affect the process and outcomes of capacity assessments (Aldous, Tomie, Worrall, & Ferguson, 2014).

People with aphasia may have intact decision-making abilities but these may be masked by receptive and expressive language difficulties (Ferguson, Duffield, & Worrall, 2010; Kagan & Kimmelman, 1995; Zuscak, Peisah, & Ferguson, 2016). There is a risk that professionals, family members and friends may erroneously conclude that a person who has aphasia lacks the ability to make a decision because their language difficulties make it more difficult for them to demonstrate their mental capacity. This is because people involved in capacity assessment who lack training in communication disorders may find it difficult to reliably identify and support communication needs (Cameron et al., 2018; Carragher et al., 2020). For example, a person with limited understanding of aphasia might assume that because an individual cannot talk about a decision (because of their expressive language difficulties), they may not understand information about the decision sufficiently to make a decision (Stein & Brady Wagner, 2006). Similarly, someone might under- or overestimate a person's ability to understand language or use "yes" and "no" reliably. An underestimation of these abilities may cause someone to conclude the person with aphasia lacks capacity when in fact they may be able to make a decision with the appropriate support. An overestimation of these abilities might lead someone to conclude the person with aphasia is able to make an informed decision, when in fact they may not, even with communication support (Kagan & Kimmelman, 1995).

Mental capacity assessments for people with aphasia and other communication disorders are, therefore, complex. As noted above, the law requires people to provide tailored decision-making support to those who require it. The ability to provide effective communication support depends on the ability to identify someone's individual communication needs. This is where we as SLTs can make an important contribution.

What is the SLT role in mental capacity assessment and supported decision-making?

Current UK mental capacity legislation clearly states that anyone 'directly concerned' with a person at the time they need to make a decision should be involved in the capacity assessment process (MCA Code of Practice, 2007, paragraph 4.38). Therefore, mental capacity assessments can be carried out by any discipline. In England and Wales, the MCA Code of Practice suggests that the mental capacity assessment process should be led by the 'decision-maker'. This is the individual (a professional, family member or friend) who will take action in a person's best interests if the capacity assessment finds that the person cannot make the decision for themselves (MCA Code of Practice, 2007, paragraph 4.42). The decision-maker needs to understand the nature of the decision the person is being asked to make, the available options, and the consequences and associated risks and benefits of each option. Therefore, a member of the medical team is likely to be the decision-maker for capacity assessments about treatment decisions. Care managers, social workers or occupational therapists (OTs) are usually the decision-makers for capacity assessments relating to care or residence decisions. Professionals with specialist financial or legal knowledge, and sometimes social workers, are usually the decision-maker when assessments involve decisions about financial arrangements or making a will. As SLTs, we can be the decision-maker for assessments involving decisions related to speech and language therapy interventions (e.g., whether to consent to an assessment or treatment) or decisions related to how to manage swallowing difficulties.

To complete a robust assessment, a mental capacity assessor needs to not only understand the nature of the decision the person is being asked to make but also how to support that person to maximize their decision-making abilities. As professionals may not have specialist knowledge of both the decision options and how to support the person to make the decision, it can be beneficial for two professionals with complementary knowledge and skills to carry out a joint assessment. Professionals have reported that they find joint assessments very useful, particularly in more complex or borderline cases, where it is not clear whether a person lacks capacity and discussion with a colleague can help to determine the outcome (Jayes, Palmer, Enderby, & Sutton, 2019).

Our training as SLTs makes us ideally placed to lead or support capacity assessments for people with communication disabilities (Volkmer, 2016; Zuscak et al., 2015). We can use our specialist knowledge and skills in assessing, diagnosing and treating communication disorders to support people with these difficulties to make decisions and demonstrate their decision-making abilities during capacity assessments. We will discuss our important role as communication facilitators when we look at practical approaches to capacity assessment later on in this chapter.

Borrett and Gould (2020) interviewed UK SLTs who work with people with aphasia about their experiences of mental capacity assessment. Their research identified a number of other roles that SLTs can play in relation to mental capacity assessment and supported decision making. Firstly, we have a key role to play in educating and training our multidisciplinary colleagues in the nature of communication disabilities and approaches to supporting communication needs. At an individual patient or service user level, this could involve completing a communication assessment and using the findings to develop practical resources and guidance for colleagues to help them support a person's communication needs during a later capacity assessment. It could also involve being present during the capacity assessment to provide and/ or model this support. At a service or team level, this could involve creating practical communication resources or delivering targeted communication training for our multidisciplinary colleagues. The value of training mental capacity assessors in communication skills was recognized by the House of Lords Select Committee that scrutinized the implementation of the MCA in England and Wales; their report commented: "…the best capacity assessments are by people…who have experience and training in communicating with people with disabilities…" (House of Lords, 2014, paragraph 69).

Volkmer (2018) provides a useful overview of models of communication training, the evidence underpinning these, and how they might be applied to mental capacity assessment and supported decision making. The Communication Aid to Capacity Evaluation (CACE) is an evidence-based training intervention designed in Canada by Carling-Rowland, Black, McDonald and Kagan (2014). CACE was designed to support social care professionals who complete capacity assessments for people with aphasia who need to make decisions about where to live and their care arrangements. It combines training in supported conversation techniques and use of specific accessible information resources. After social work professionals received this training, their communication skills improved, they completed more accurate mental capacity assessments, and they felt more confident about their practice. Importantly, the people with aphasia reported they felt they were better able to communicate with the professionals and felt less frustrated during the capacity assessments after staff had been trained. More information on CACE is available here: https://www.aphasia.ca/home-page/health-care-professionals/resources-and-tools/cace/

As SLTs, we have an important and multifaceted role to play in mental capacity assessment and supported decision making. This is recognized in the international literature (e.g., Aldous et al., 2014; Ferguson et al., 2010; Suleman & Hopper, 2015). In the UK, the SLT role is promoted by the RCSLT (2018), the General Medical Council (2020), the MCA Code of Practice (DCA, 2007), the AISA Code of Practice (Scottish Government, 2010), and the NICE guideline on decision-making and mental capacity (NG108; NICE, 2018). However, it still appears that our role may not be understood or recognized by some professionals. In some settings, perceived professional hierarchies appear to determine who assesses capacity: particular disciplines and more senior staff members tend to lead assessments (Jayes et al., 2019). In other settings, healthcare staff may not be aware that SLTs have specialist skills in communication assessment and inclusive communication methods that can be used to facilitate decision making (McCormick et al., 2017), or that we have the resources to be involved in capacity assessments (Jayes, Palmer, & Enderby, 2017). It is therefore key that we attempt as a profession and as individual practitioners to educate our colleagues about the contribution we can make to mental capacity assessment and supported decision-making.

What does a mental capacity assessment involve?

As noted above, if somebody who is involved in the care of a person with aphasia has reason to believe that the person may have difficulty making a particular decision, then they should consider completing a mental capacity assessment. In order to be valid, the assessment should be completed at the time the decision needs to be made. Capacity assessments are usually conducted using a conversation format during semi-structured clinical interviews (Emmett, Pool, Bond, & Hughes, 2013; Suleman & Hopper, 2015). During these conversations, assessors provide information to patients or service users (service user here denotes anyone who accesses health or social care services) about the decisions they are being asked to make and the options available to them.

Unfortunately, there is currently no established gold standard tool to help SLTs carry out mental capacity assessments. Although assessment tools do exist, these tend to be based on legal frameworks outside the UK and do not enable assessors to meet the needs of people with communication difficulties. For more information about these tools, see Lamont, Jeon and Chiarella (2013), and Pennington, Davey, Meulen, Coulthard and Kehoe (2018). In the absence of any gold standard measure, a number of sources of evidence provide useful suggestions for best practice in UK mental capacity assessment. These include the Mental Capacity Act Code of Practice (2007), the House of Lords Select Committee Report (2014), the NICE Guideline NG108 (2018), and a review of the literature and case law relating to mental capacity assessment practice in England and Wales (Jayes et al., 2019). Although these sources of evidence relate to the legal framework for England and Wales, the practice guidance they provide is likely to be useful to SLTs working in Northern Ireland and Scotland. The following sections provide a synthesis of this evidence.

Before the assessment: Preparation

Before starting the capacity assessment with the patient or service user, the assessor(s) should engage in comprehensive preparation work, to ensure the assessment process is legally robust and the person is fully supported to maximise their decision-making abilities. It is important to collect different types of information to inform the assessment. These are shown in Table 5.2.

All this information can be used to plan how to provide information about the decision during the capacity assessment and support the person to understand and use it to make a decision. It is important to identify what relevant information the person would need in order to be able to make the particular decision. Assessors should take care not to give patients or service users overly complex, technical information or information that involves specialist language; this is particularly important when assessing people with aphasia and other communication disorders.

When planning the capacity assessment, it is good practice to select a physical environment that will support the person to maximize their decision-making abilities. For people with communication and/or cognitive difficulties, it is helpful to try to minimize visual and auditory distractions and to ensure that the space is well lit and comfortable. It is also important to consider how fatigue or medication effects may impact on the person's ability to engage in a conversation and in decision making and to plan the timing and duration of the capacity assessment to mitigate for these. If the person has any sensory needs, these should be addressed prior to commencing the capacity assessment.

Table 5.2 Information to collect in preparation for a capacity assessment.

Type of information	Questions you need to answer	Where to find this information
Information about the person being assessed	• What health condition does the person have that could cause difficulties with decision making: what is the impairment or disturbance of their mind or brain? • Is the impairment or disturbance caused by a temporary condition (e.g., due to a delirium)? In this case, consider delaying the capacity assessment until these difficulties have resolved. If this is not possible, review the person's ability to make the decision at a later date. • What are their decision-making support needs? Do they have cognitive or communication needs? Do they have emotional or mental health needs? • How are these needs best supported during a capacity assessment, and by whom? • How does the person normally approach decision-making (e.g., do they like to involve their family or friends)? • Have they made any advance care plans that relate to this decision?	• Ask the person. • Check if they have a communication passport. • Look for information in their care record. • Check how they manage on assessments of relevant abilities (e.g., communication). • Ask family members or care professionals about their observations.
Information about the decision	• What is the specific decision? • Why does the person need to make the decision? • What are the available decision options? • What are the benefits, risks, likely consequences of each option? • What happens if the person does not make the decision? • What is the timescale for decision-making? • Who would be the decision-maker if the person is found to lack capacity?	• Look for information in their care record. • Talk to the multidisciplinary team.

For example, the assessor(s) should ensure the person is wearing glasses or a hearing aid if they need them and that they have well-fitting dentures if they need these to speak clearly and comfortably.

It is advisable to explain in advance to the person what the assessment will involve in order to prepare them for the conversation. Some patients or service users may be apprehensive about discussing important decisions with health and social care professionals. For this reason, it may beneficial to ask someone familiar (e.g., a family member or a carer who knows the person well) to be present during the assessment to offer reassurance. Even if they do not feel they need reassurance, some patients and service users may appreciate the opportunity to discuss a decision with family members or friends. This is particular likely if the potential consequences of the decision have implications for family members (e.g., a change of residence or care arrangements).

Some patients may not be used to making significant decisions without people from their family or their local community being present. As noted earlier, UK mental capacity legislation is based on Western ethical frameworks that value personal autonomy and self-determination (Chettif, 2012). These frameworks promote a very individualistic approach to decision making. However, some cultural groups approach decision making in more collective ways. Hawley and Morris (2017) provide a helpful overview of issues relating to culture and decision making. It is therefore important to ask the patient or service user if they would like a family member or friend to be present during the assessment. If any such people attend the assessment, it is beneficial to provide a clear explanation beforehand of the purpose of the assessment, what will happen during it, and the role they can play in it.

Supporting decision-making

As noted previously, UK mental capacity legislation requires assessors to provide whatever type of support people need to understand, think and communicate about decisions. As SLTs, we should be familiar with and skilled in supporting people's communication needs. The type of communication support required by each person during a capacity assessment will depend on that individual's specific needs but is likely to involve a combination of inclusive communication approaches. Examples of inclusive communication approaches are shown in Figure 5.3. It is important also to consider how to support the communication needs of people who speak English as a second language or who have hearing or visual disabilities. In these situations, guidance and practical support should

- Use the person's preferred communication method.

- Use simple, everyday words.

- Use short, simple sentences (1 main idea per sentence).

- Speak slowly and clearly and give the person extra time.

- Use and encourage the person to use total communication strategies (e.g., writing, gesture, drawing) and communication aids (alphabet chart, visual scales, photos, Talking Mats ©, electronic aids).

- If using written language, adopt accessible or 'aphasia-friendly' information guidelines (e.g., Herbert et al., 2012). For more information about this, see Jayes (2018).

- Introduce changes in topic to structure the conversation.

- Repeat key information/recap.

- Check the person's understanding as you go along.

- Take regular breaks to avoid fatigue.

Figure 5.3 Examples of inclusive communication approaches.

be sought from specialist interpreters. A set of practical resources has been specifically developed to support capacity assessments for hospital patients with communication disabilities (Allen and Bryer, 2014).

People with cognitive difficulties (e.g., those who find it hard to attend to and/or retain information) also require tailored support during capacity assessments. Some SLTs may have skills in supporting people with these types of difficulty; for those who do not, it is important to seek specialist support from multidisciplinary colleagues such as an occupational therapist, psychologist or mental health professional. Suleman and Kim (2015) provide a helpful overview of how cognitive difficulties can impact on the process of mental capacity assessment, and how such difficulties might be supported. Similarly, patients or service users may have mental health conditions that could affect their ability to communicate and think about decisions. In this situation, capacity assessors may need to recruit assistance from mental health professionals or SLT colleagues with specialist skills in working with people with mental health conditions.

The nature of the impairment/disturbance of the mind or brain.

The reasons why the person is able or unable to make the decision.

The practicable steps taken to help the person make the decision.

The outcome of the assessment and reasons for this conclusion.

If the person is found to lack capacity, the fact that their inability to make a decision is a direct consequence of the impairment or disturbance.

Why the assessor considers this an incapacitous decision rather than an unwise one.

Figure 5.4 Suggested information to include in a record of a mental capacity assessment.

Testing decision-making abilities

When information has been provided about the decision and options available, the assessor needs to determine whether the person can understand, retain and use this information in order to make a decision. Table 5.1 provides more information about the requirements of the legal functional test of decision making in each UK jurisdiction. Assessors tend to ask people questions in order to test their decision-making abilities. For example, to ascertain how much information somebody understands and remembers about the decision, the assessor(s) could ask open questions such as "Why do you think you need to make this decision?" or "What are the different options available to you?" To assess someone's ability to use or weigh the information, the assessor(s) could ask "Why is this decision important?", "What are the pros and cons of deciding to do that?", or "Why have you chosen that option?" When asking any patient or service user such questions, it is essential to use simple, non-technical and non-judgemental language, and to avoid asking leading questions. Capacity assessors need to remain neutral about decision options, even though some patients or service users may want to know what the professional would do in their position.

For people with cognitive and communicative difficulties, it is important to adjust the way these decision-making abilities are tested in order to support individuals to demonstrate their capacity in whatever way they can. In this situation, SLTs are practised in using inclusive communication approaches and other techniques to reduce the complexity of language or information processing load when asking questions. For example, it is possible to ask simple closed questions or 'forced alternatives' to check people's understanding and retention of key facts. Use of written language and images may support people who have difficulties understanding and using spoken language. For example, the assessor(s) could ask a patient or service user to write down their answer to a question or select and point to the written answer or an image representing the same concept from a number of distractors. In addition, the assessor(s) could ask the person to sort images corresponding to different concepts (e.g., the pros and cons of different decision options) into piles to demonstrate their ability to understand, retain, and use and weigh information.

Documentation

As for any intervention with a patient or service user, a mental capacity assessment requires contemporaneous, clear and legible documentation. The Mental Capacity Act Code of Practice (2007) and NICE guideline NG108 (2018) suggest that records of capacity assessments should include the information shown in Figure 5.4. Local organizations are likely to have their own policies relating to documentation and many have developed their own proformas to support staff in documenting capacity assessments. There is evidence to suggest that assessors appreciate documentation aids and that these can lead to improvements in documentation quality (Emmett et al., 2013; Jayes, Palmer, & Enderby, 2020; Ramasubramanian, Ranasinghe, & Ellison, 2011).

Capacity assessment: A challenging area of practice

Completing a robust capacity assessment and determining whether or not an individual lacks the ability to make a potentially life-changing decision for themselves, even with support, can be challenging. As suggested above, the process requires comprehensive preparation and close liaison with other professionals, patients or service users, their family members, friends and carers. It also requires specialist knowledge and skills. In the absence of any gold standard assessment tool, the process of identifying that a person lacks capacity fundamentally relies on subjective judgements. Furthermore, the outcomes of capacity assessments can have important implications for the people we work with and their families; these outcomes may limit individuals' abilities to retain independent control of many aspects of their daily lives (Lamont et al., 2013). In addition to this, our assessment processes may be examined by regulatory bodies or subject to legal scrutiny.

Perhaps unsurprisingly, then, evidence from the UK (McCormick et al., 2017) and overseas (Aldous et al., 2014) suggests that SLTs find mental capacity work demanding and feel under-confident about their practice. We are not alone in this, as other disciplines have reported similar feelings (Jayes et al., 2017; Willner, Bridle, Price, Dymond, & Lewis, 2013). Research evidence and case law also suggest that some aspects of current practice are not consistent with legal requirements and patients and service users may not always receive the opportunities or support they need to engage in decision-making (House of Lords, 2014; Jayes et al., 2019).

In response to these challenges, the NICE guideline NG108 (2018) recommends that evidence-based training and tools should be developed to enable assessors to improve their practice and gain confidence. Until these become available, we can engage in a number of activities to help us develop our skills and confidence. As for any aspect of our work, we should endeavour to reflect on our mental capacity practice, through individual supervision or mentoring and case discussion with colleagues. We should consider auditing our assessment documentation in order to identify targets for improvement. We can learn relevant practical skills by accessing training or by observing colleagues during assessments. Finally, searching the emerging evidence base and participating in professional networks of SLTs engaged in this work can enable us to identify and share new practice developments.

Conclusion

This chapter has introduced the concept of mental capacity and the different UK legal frameworks that safeguard the rights of people to make autonomous decisions and receive decision-making support tailored to their individual needs. For people with communication disorders such as aphasia, the legislation emphasizes the need for person-centred communication support. SLTs therefore have both an ethical and a legal responsibility to ensure the people we work with have opportunities and effective support to make decisions, or at least have their voices heard when decisions are made about them. This chapter has also provided suggestions for how SLTs new to mental capacity assessment should approach this work, based on best practice recommendations from current guidance and research evidence. Although mental capacity work can be challenging and resource-intensive, SLTs' expertise in assessing and supporting the needs of people with communication disorders means that we have a range of important roles to play in this growing area of interdisciplinary practice and a unique skill set to enable us to fulfil these roles.

References

Aldous, K., Tolmie, R., Worrall, L., & Ferguson, A. (2014). Speech-language pathologists' contribution to the assessment of decision-making capacity in aphasia: A survey of common practices. *International Journal of Speech-Language Pathology*, 16, 231-241.

Allen, J. & Bryer, H. (2014). Supporting adults with communication impairment to make decisions. Available from: http://www.blacksheeppress.co.uk/products/adults/MCA#

Bailey, D. (2018). The mental capacity legislation across England and Wales, Scotland and Northern Ireland: Relevance to healthcare. In I. Jones & A. Volkmer (Eds), *Speech and Language Therapists and Mental Capacity: A Training Resource for Adult Services*, pp.1-24. Guildford: J&R Press.

Beauchamp, T.L. & Childress, J.F. (2008). *Principles of Biomedical Ethics*, 6th ed. Oxford, UK: OUP.

Borrett, S. & Gould, L.J. (2020). Mental capacity assessment with people with aphasia: Understanding the role of the speech and language therapist. *Aphasiology*. https://doi.org/10.1080/02687038.2020.1819954

Cameron, A., McPhail, S., Hudson, K., Fleming, J., Lethlean, J., Tan, N.J., & Finch, E. (2018). The confidence and knowledge of health practitioners when interacting with people with aphasia in a hospital setting. *Disability and Rehabilitation*, 40(11), 1288-1293.

Carling-Rowland, A., Black, S., McDonald, L., & Kagan, A. (2014). Increasing access to fair capacity evaluation for discharge decision-making for people with aphasia: A randomised controlled trial. *Aphasiology*, 28(6), 750-765.

Carragher, M., Steel, G., O'Halloran, R., Torabi, T., Johnson, H., Taylor, N.F., & Rose, M. (2020). Aphasia disrupts usual care: The stroke team's perceptions of delivering healthcare to patients with aphasia. *Disability and Rehabilitation*. https://doi.org/10.1080/09638288.2020.1722264

Chettif, M. (2012). Turning the lens inward: Cultural competence and providers' values in health care decision making. *The Gerontologist*, 52(6), 739-747.

Department of Constitutional Affairs (2007). *Mental Capacity Act Code of Practice*. London: Department of Constitutional Affairs.

Elwyn, G. et al. (2012). Shared decision making: A model for clinical practice. *Journal of General Internal Medicine*, 27(10), 1361-1367.

Emmett, C., Poole, M., Bond., J., & Hughes, J.C. (2013). Homeward bound or bound for a home? Assessing the capacity of dementia patients to make decisions about hospital discharge: Comparing practice with legal standards. *International Journal of Law and Psychiatry*, 36, 73-82.

Ferguson, A., Duffield, G., & Worrall, L. (2010). Legal decision-making by people with aphasia: Critical incidents for speech pathologists. *International Journal of Language and Communication Disorders*, 45(2), 244-268.

General Medical Council (2020). Decision making and consent [online]. Manchester, General Medical Council. Available from: https://www.gmc-uk.org/ethical-guidance/ ethical-guidance-for-doctors/decision-making-and-consent

Hawley, S.T. & Morris, A.M. (2017) Cultural challenges to engaging patients in shared decision making. *Patient Education and Counseling*, 100(1), 18–24.

Herbert, R., Haw, C., Brown C., Gregory, E., & Brumfitt, S. (2012). Stroke Association Accessible Information Guidelines. Available from: http://www.stroke.org.uk/sites/ default/files/Accessible%20Information%20Guidelines.pdf.pdf

House of Lords Select Committee on the Mental Capacity Act 2005 (2014). Mental Capacity Act 2005: Post-legislative scrutiny, HL (2013-14) 139. Available from: https://publications. parliament.uk/pa/ld201314/ldselect/ldmentalcap/139/13902.htm

Jayes, M. (2018). Supporting multidisciplinary colleagues to develop and use accessible written information materials during capacity assessments. In I. Jones & A. Volkmer (Eds), *Speech and Language Therapists and Mental Capacity: A Training Resource for Adult Services* (pp.201-221). Guildford: J&R Press.

Jayes, M., Palmer, R., & Enderby, P. (2017). An exploration of mental capacity assessment within acute hospital and intermediate care. *Disability and Rehabilitation*, 39(21), 2148-2157. https://doi.org/10.1080/09638288.2016.1224275

Jayes, M., Palmer, R. & Enderby, P. (2020). Evaluation of the MCAST, a multidisciplinary toolkit to improve mental capacity assessment. *Disability and Rehabilitation*. https:// doi.org/10.1080/09638288.2020.1765030.

Jayes, M., Palmer, R., Enderby, P., & Sutton, A. (2019). How do health and social care professionals in England and Wales assess mental capacity? A literature review. *Disability and Rehabilitation*. ttps://doi.org/10.1080/09638288.2019.1572793

Kagan, A. & Kimmelman, M. (1995). Informed consent in aphasia research: Myth or reality? *Clinical Aphasiology*, 23, 65-75.

Kim, E.S., Suleman, S., & Hopper, T. (2020). Decision making by people with aphasia: A comparison of linguistic and nonlinguistic measures. *Journal of Speech, Language, and Hearing Research*, 63(6), 1845-1860.

Lamont, S., Jeon, Y-H., & Chiarella, M. (2013). Assessing patient capacity to consent to treatment: An integrative review of instruments and tools. *Journal of Clinical Nursing*, 22(17-18) 2387-2403.

McCormick, M., Bose, A., & Marinis T. (2017). Decision-making capacity in aphasia: SLT's contribution in England. *Aphasiology*, 31(11), 1344-1358.

Murrell, A. & McCalla, L. (2016). Assessing decision-making capacity: The interpretation and implementation of the Mental Capacity Act 2005 amongst social care professionals. *Practice: Social Work in Action*, 28, 21–26.

National Institute for Health and Care Excellence (2018). Decision-making and mental capacity [NICE guideline NG108] [online] Available from: http://www.nice.org.uk/ guidance/ng108

NHS England Accessible Information Standard (2015). Available from: https://www.england. nhs.uk/ourwork/accessibleinfo/

Office of Public Sector Information (2005) *Mental Capacity Act 2005*. London: OPSI.

Pennington, C., Davey, K., Meulen, R.T., Coulthard, E., & Kehoe, P.G. (2018) Tools for testing decision-making capacity in dementia. *Age and Ageing*, 47, 778-784.

Ramasubramanian, L., Ranasinghe, N., & Ellison, J. (2011). Evaluation of a structured assessment framework to enable adherence to the requirements of Mental Capacity Act 2005. *British Journal of Learning Disabilities*, 39, 314-20.

RCSLT (2018). Position statement: The unique and essential contribution of speech and language therapists to supported decision making and mental capacity assessment [online]. Available from: https://www.rcslt.org/-/media/Project/RCSLT/rcslt-position-statement-supported-decision-making-and-mental-capacity.pdf

Seedhouse, D. (2009). *Ethics: The Heart of Health Care*, 3rd ed. Chichester, UK: Wiley-Blackwell.

Stein, J. & Brady Wagner, L. (2006). Is informed consent a "yes or no" response? Enhancing the shared decision-making process for persons with aphasia. *Topics in Stroke Rehabilitation*, 13(4), 42-46.

Suleman, S. & Hopper, T. (2015). Decision-making capacity and aphasia: Speech-language pathologists' perspectives. *Aphasiology*. doi: 10.1080/02687038.2015.1065468

Suleman, S. & Kim, E. (2015). Decision-making, cognition, and aphasia: Developing a foundation for future discussions and inquiry. *Aphasiology*. doi: 10.1080/02687038.2012.1049584

The British Psychological Society (BPS) (2010). *Audit Tool for Mental Capacity Assessments*. Leicester: The British Psychological Society.

The Scottish Government (2008). *Adults with Incapacity (Scotland) Act 2000*. Edinburgh: The Scottish Government.

The Scottish Government (2010). *Adults with Incapacity (Scotland) Act 2000 Code of Practice (Third Edition)*. Edinburgh: The Scottish Government.

The Stationery Office (2016). Mental Capacity Act (Northern Ireland). Norwich: The Stationary Office. Available from: https://www.legislation.gov.uk/nia/2016/18/contents/enacted

Volkmer, A. (2016). Advance care planning: Supporting people to plan for their future as a speech and language therapist. In A. Volkmer (Ed.), *Dealing with Capacity and Other Legal Issues with Adults with Acquired Neurological Conditions*, pp.163-184. Guildford: J&R Press.

Volkmer, A. (2018). Communication skills training to support decision making. In I. Jones & A. Volkmer (Eds) *Speech and Language Therapists and Mental Capacity: A Training Resource for Adult Services*, pp.165-199. Guildford: J&R Press.

Willner, P., Bridle, J., Price, V., Dymond, S., & Lewis, G. (2013). What do NHS staff learn from training on the Mental Capacity Act (2005)? *Legal and Criminological Psychology*, 18, 83-101.

Zuscak, S.J., Peisah, C., & Ferguson, A. (2016). A collaborative approach to supporting communication in the assessment of decision making capacity. *Disability & Rehabilitation*, 38(11), 1107-1114.

6 Psychological Wellbeing in Aphasia

Eirini Kontou, Shirley Thomas and Posy Knights

Introduction

Stroke usually has a sudden onset and can lead to impairment of sensory, motor, cognitive and communication abilities. It can severely impact a person's emotions both at the time of the stroke but also in the months and years that follow (Stroke Association, 2019). Anxiety has been reported up to 10 years (Ayerbe, Ayis, Crichton, Wolfe, & Rudd, 2014) and depression up to 15 years post-stroke (Ayerbe, Ayis, Crichton, Wolfe, & Rudd, 2013). Depression, followed by anxiety, are the most commonly investigated psychological consequences of stroke and have negative impacts on rehabilitation outcomes, carer strain and mortality (Lincoln, Kneebone, Macniven, & Morris, 2012). Systematic reviews report that about one-third of people have depression at any time point following stroke (Ayerbe et al., 2013; Hackett & Pickles, 2014), with rates of anxiety reported between 18.7% and 24.2% (Knapp et al., 2020). People can also experience psychological impact or distress which is not severe enough to meet criteria for a clinical diagnosis but which can still have negative effects on the individual and their life (Thomas, Walker, Macniven, Haworth, & Lincoln, 2013).

Aphasia can impact upon all areas of a person's life, including personal, professional, social and family. People with aphasia may be particularly at risk of depression (Kauhanen et al., 2000) and anxiety (Morris et al., 2017b), and the presence (Åström, Adolfsson, & Asplund, 1993) and severity (Thomas & Lincoln, 2008) of communication impairment have been found to be predictors of distress after stroke. Previously, people with aphasia have typically been excluded from studies assessing (Townend, Brady, & McLaughlan, 2007) and treating depression (Baker et al., 2017) or anxiety (Knapp et al., 2020) following stroke. Many studies do not explicitly report whether people with aphasia were included.

This chapter outlines the importance of addressing aspects of psychological wellbeing following stroke, from assessment to management, for enabling people with aphasia to access meaningful support. It is primarily aimed at speech and language therapists and it features examples that cover a wide range of therapeutic models. We provide here an overview of practical techniques that can be considered when supporting people with aphasia and their families.

Assessing psychological wellbeing in people with aphasia

The National Clinical Guideline for Stroke (RCP, 2016) recommends that mood should be screened within six weeks of stroke and at six and 12 months, and that people with one mood disorder (e.g. depression) should be assessed for others (e.g., anxiety). It is outside the scope of this chapter to present a comprehensive review of mood assessments for people with aphasia as relevant systematic reviews have been published (e.g., van Dijk, de Man-van Ginkel, Hafsteinsdóttir, & Schuurmans, 2016). This chapter will focus on depression and anxiety as these have been the most commonly researched, but the principles of choosing an assessment could apply to other domains.

Symptoms of depression and anxiety are typically identified using a questionnaire or a clinical interview. It can be helpful to consider the symptoms along a continuum rather than a clinical diagnosis. It is relevant to consider the purpose of the assessment as this will influence the psychometric and practical properties you would look for. Assessments can be used for screening, more in-depth assessment, or monitoring change. Screening assessments, usually a questionnaire, are completed with a large number of people with the aim to identify, using a cut-off score, people who may have depression or anxiety and where more detailed assessment is then needed. Assessments, usually a clinical interview, can also be used to diagnose people as having anxiety or depression.

When choosing a mood assessment you should consider psychometric properties, namely reliability and validity, and, where relevant, the accuracy of the cut-off score for identifying symptoms of depression or anxiety. A key point is that the psychometric properties should be evaluated in the clinical group who it is to be used with (e.g., post-stroke aphasia). There are also practical factors. Screening assessments should be short and simple so they can be used with a large number of people. Consideration should be given to the cognitive demands of an assessment (e.g., memory, attention, concentration) and physical requests (e.g., point at a stimulus). Depending on the context of your service, you may also need to consider cost, ease of scoring and whether any training is needed.

Most standardized mood assessments rely on the individual to be able to communicate adequately (van Dijk et al., 2016). Few mood screening questionnaires have been developed and evaluated specifically for people with aphasia. Mood screening should be part of a pathway which would include follow-up assessment and intervention for those identified as having difficulties. Some people with aphasia are able to complete the same self-report questionnaire as people without aphasia. Adapted self-report questionnaires have been designed to use with people with aphasia, in particular picture-based or visual analogue assessments.

Examples of visual analogue scales:

- Depression Intensity Scale Circles (DISCS; Turner-Stokes, Kalmus, Hirani, & Clegg, 2005): A short and simple single-item scale depicting six circles which have an increased amount of grey shading as you move from the bottom to the top circle. Designed for using with people who have communication and/or cognitive problems following brain injury. Freely available from: https://www.kcl.ac.uk/cicelysaunders/resources/tools/discs

- Visual Analog Mood Scale (VAMS; Stern, 1997) and Visual Analog Mood Scale-Revised (VAMS-R; Kontou, Thomas, & Lincoln, 2012): Developed for people with neurological conditions. Eight-item scale consisting of stimuli and line drawings of faces and a single word presented at the top and bottom of a 10cm vertical line.

- Visual Analogue Self-Esteem Scale (VASES; Brumfitt & Sheeran, 1999): Designed to assess self-esteem in people with communication impairments but includes a depression item. Each item is a stimulus card with a pair of line drawings and a response scale below. There are no published cut-offs for depression screening but may be useful for indicating severity and monitoring change (Bennett, Thomas, Austen, Morris, & Lincoln, 2006).

- Dynamic Visual Analogue Mood Scales (D-VAMS; Barrows & Thomas, 2018): Recently developed assessment consisting of photographs of facial expressions which are modulated via a slide control on a tablet/computer. Available from: http://www.dvams.com/dvams/about.aspx

An alternative or adjunct to a self-report questionnaire is an observer-rated (or proxy) measure. This is a questionnaire completed by someone else (e.g., staff on a stroke ward, a partner or relative if in the community) to assess depression or anxiety based on observable behaviours. However, self-reported information remains an important source of information. A systematic review (van Dijk et al., 2016) recommended the Stroke Aphasic Depression Questionnaire (SADQ-10; Sutcliffe & Lincoln, 1998), the Stroke Aphasic Depression Questionnaire-Hospital 10 (SADQH-10H; Lincoln, Sutcliffe, & Unsworth, 2000) and the Signs of Depression Scale (SOD; Watkins et al., 2001) for screening depression in people with aphasia in clinical practice. The Behavioural Outcomes of Anxiety Scale (BOA; Eccles, Morris, & Kneebone, 2017) has been developed for screening symptoms of anxiety and has been validated in people with aphasia.

Psychological therapies and aphasia

Over the past two decades, there is increasing evidence for the application of a range of therapeutic approaches for supporting stroke survivors, including those with aphasia problems (Meredith & Yeates, 2020; Baker et al., 2018).

Cognitive Behavioural Therapy (CBT) refers to a wide range of approaches that are often synonymous with evidence-based practice irrespective of the strength of evidence or the clinical challenges that may be presented when working with people with aphasia. Modification and individual tailoring of CBT is likely to be needed to accommodate cognitive and communication difficulties where these are experienced following stroke (Kneebone, 2016). For example, in a framework to support CBT for emotional disorders following stroke, Kneebone (2016) suggests that as cognitive and communication difficulties become more prominent, treatment is likely to focus on behavioural elements such as behavioural activation for depression.

A specific form of 'CBT' practice when working with people with aphasia is behavioural activation (BA). Other approaches, such as Mindfulness Based Cognitive Therapy (MBCT), Acceptance and Commitment Therapy (ACT) and Compassion Focused Therapy (CFT) can share common components that are more focused on the *context* and *processes* of how a person relates to internal experiences (e.g., thoughts, emotions, physical sensations). In this chapter, we will focus on the basic principles and how these approaches can be informally used to promote psychological wellbeing in the context of people who experience aphasia.

From a practical perspective, it is important to highlight the role of partners, family members and friends for any of these psychological interventions. This not only acknowledges the important role of significant others in the recovery journey after stroke, but also highlights the need to consider contraindications or how certain approaches may be more challenging for people with severe aphasia. This also resonates with our professional reflections on using a wide range of psychologically informed therapies that are adapted based on the lived experiences of stroke survivors and their individual needs.

What is Behavioural Activation?

An intervention approach which can be adapted to be accessible for people with aphasia is Behavioural Activation (BA). BA is based on the behavioural model of depression whereby depression is thought to result from a lack of response-contingent positive reinforcement (Lewinsohn, 1974). Response-contingent positive reinforcement means that a person's actions have pleasant or positive consequences so they are more likely to repeat those actions in the future (e.g., being praised for completing a task, or self-reinforcement where an individual rewards or congratulates themselves). Low positive reinforcement can arise from reduced availability of reinforcers in the environment (such as having less contact with people who might give you praise or compliments), insufficiency in skills (such as social skills) and decreased ability to enjoy activities. Stroke and aphasia can bring about a reduction in rewarding activities and interactions (including everyday activities, hobbies, social contacts). As an individual's mood becomes low they may further withdraw from engaging in activities, and the situation becomes a vicious cycle. BA aims to increase the level of activity, particularly for valued or positively reinforcing events, and reduce avoidance behaviours to improve mood. An example of an avoidance behaviour is avoiding meeting a friend because of finding the social contact difficult.

BA has been found to be effective at treating depression in adults in primary care (Mazzucchelli, Kane, & Rees, 2009) and older adults (Scogin, Welsh, Hanson, Stump, & Coates, 2005) and has comparable effectiveness to CBT (Cuijpers et al., 2013; Richards et al., 2016). There is some indication that BA is beneficial at treating depression in neurological conditions (Oates, Moghaddam, Evangelou, & das Nair, 2020). BA could be applicable to people with aphasia because it is a relatively straightforward and practical approach, does not require a highly trained therapist and can be adapted to accommodate communication impairments. A multicentre randomized controlled trial (RCT) evaluating BA delivered by an assistant psychologist for treating low mood in people with post-stroke aphasia found that mood was significantly better at 6-month follow-up in those who received BA compared with those receiving usual care (Thomas et al., 2013). BA has also been found to be feasible for treating post-stroke depression in people with and without aphasia or with cognitive impairment, and therapy was acceptable to participants, carers and therapists (Thomas et al., 2019).

The BA approaches used in these studies are outlined in this chapter. Individualized goals are agreed with the client which focus on increasing enjoyable or valued activities. Broadly, the BA programme in these studies involved finding out how the individual spends their time, identifying activities they enjoy engaging in (including resuming previous activities, increasing current activities and starting new activities) and increasing the level of valued activities.

An overview of key BA techniques:

- **Activity monitoring**: Find out how individuals are spending their time and their current activity levels. This can be done using an activity diary and the complexity of the diary can be adapted for the communication and cognitive abilities of the person. Reviewing the diary with the individual can also help see changes over time. In addition, individuals can record mood ratings for their enjoyment of an activity or a day to explore how the value of activities may relate to mood.

- **Activity scheduling**: Identify activities the individual values then plan in advance realistic activities and goals for each day. This gives a structure to the day and removes 'on the spot' decision making and avoidance. Activities are individualized based on abilities and goals. The aim is to gradually increase activity levels and therefore positive reinforcement to improve mood. A similar format to the activity monitoring diary can be used for activity scheduling.

- **Graded tasks**: Breaking down a large task into smaller manageable steps to facilitate practice and making difficult tasks more achievable. This increases opportunity for self-reward (such as self-praise for achieving each step) and reducing avoidance (where attempting the large task at the outset can seem daunting). An example was a lady with aphasia who used to go to the local town alone on the bus but had lost confidence since her stroke. The first step in the graded task was going with her daughter on the bus to town for a short visit, followed by a longer visit with a friend, then going on her own to meet her daughter or friend and ending with going on the bus to town and back on her own.

- **Between-session tasks**: Tasks to complete between sessions are integral to BA. For example, at the beginning of therapy this might be completing an activity diary while later tasks could include practising graded tasks.

- **Problem solving**: Difficulties with completing activities or between-session tasks should be identified. Reasons might include not having time, forgetting, low motivation, or the task being too difficult. Problem solving can be used to find solutions to difficulties by brainstorming possible solutions and discussing the pros and cons of each to choose which to try out.

Figure 6.1 summarizes ways in which BA can be adapted to use with people with aphasia.

Participants who received BA for post-stroke depression were interviewed about their experiences and highlighted the value of breaking down bigger tasks and reviewing their progress (Thomas et al., 2019).

> "You try to do things and you struggle because […] you're not cutting the picture down, you're just trying to look at the whole thing. But this encourages you to break things down into little bits, rather than the whole thing, which is a better way of doing it."

Record key points during the session, e.g., using a notebook.

Adjust the format of the activity diary or schedule for the individual's communication abilities and preferences.

Record between-session tasks in an accessible format.

Summarize and check understanding during and at the end of a session.

Utilize communication resources that a person already finds helpful. This might include pen and paper for writing key words and drawing, using pictures and photos, etc.

Figure 6.1 Adapting BA for people with post-stroke aphasia.

"And I think that's something that I realised during the sort of weekly reflections, that that's the life attitude that really fights off downs. You know, my really giving myself a pat on the back for what I have done, rather than concentrating on what I can't do."

From our experience, behavioural activation may be particularly relevant for working with individuals where their cognitive and/or communication difficulties mean a more concrete and practical approach is helpful and also for individuals where low mood may be associated with low activity levels.

Mindfulness-based interventions

Mindfulness has become a buzzword and there are several popular definitions. It is often used as a term to describe standalone meditation approaches for staying in the present moment and 'being mindful' of one's thoughts or feelings. Mindfulness refers to paying attention to thoughts, sounds, emotions, or physical sensations in a non-judgemental way with the aim of bringing the attention back to the present moment whenever the mind starts to wander. Contrary to popular belief, mindfulness is not a relaxation technique but, when practised, it can lead to feelings of calm and relaxation.

Mindfulness-Based Stress Reduction (MBSR) was developed by Jon Kabat-Zinn in the 1980s and Mindfulness-Based Cognitive Therapy (MBCT) is an adaptation of MBSR that uses the same basic format and structure to combine mindfulness and CBT techniques. Evidence is building on the use of mindfulness-based interventions (largely from MBSR) in helping people with neurological conditions to cope better with symptoms of anxiety and depression (McLean, Lawrence, Simpson, & Mercer, 2017; Simpson et al., 2014; Wood, Lawrence, Jani, Simpson, & Mercer, 2017).

The application of mindfulness in stroke recovery is supported by few studies. In a systematic review of mindfulness-based interventions (MBIs) for stroke survivors, Lawrence and colleagues (2013) proposed a range of physiological and psychosocial benefits for managing anxiety, depression, mental fatigue, and improvements in overall quality of life. To date, evidence as to the effectiveness of mindfulness for stroke survivors with aphasia has been shown in a number of small case studies (Dickinson, Friary, & McCann, 2016; Panda, Whitworth, Hersh, & Biedermann, 2020; Orenstein, Basilakos, & Marshall, 2012).

MBIs can be delivered flexibly and in different formats (individual and/ or group sessions) to support the psychological wellbeing of people with communication problems. What is often particularly relevant about the approaches and techniques described here is that they can be applicable to a wide range of presenting difficulties. Mindfulness can be considered not only as a way to improve mood but also other stroke-related difficulties such as pain or fatigue.

Although these psychological approaches can be delivered by qualified and trained psychological practitioners they can also be employed by other healthcare professionals with appropriate training and supervision. The observations and therapeutic work completed by Speech and Language Therapy are critical in supporting the delivery of practical sessions that can be adapted to introduce the concept of mindfulness and to incorporate simple exercises. To this end, two example practices are presented here.

Examples of mindfulness exercises

Wang and colleagues (2019) reported on stroke survivors' preferred mindfulness and relaxation techniques, including suggestions on adaptations and practice frequency. Mardula and Vaughn (2020) describe personal reflections and simple mindfulness techniques that were adapted and used by a mindfulness expert when she herself became a stroke survivor.

Typically consider a short exercise such as breathing space or body scan lasting one to five minutes. Here are two simple examples that can be used to introduce mindfulness ideas and to encourage focus on the 'here and now'.

Exploring what works best for the person, practising together in a session and asking how they feel after a practice can help to determine the benefits of practising these exercises. Encourage regular practice, and support the person to find the exercises that are most helpful to them when adjusting to life after stroke.

- **Example Practice 1: Breathing space**

  Sit down on a chair or you can choose to lie down.

  Try to find a comfortable position.

  Close your eyes if that feels OK with you.

  Become aware of your breath around the area of your belly.

  Breathe in through your nose and breathe out through your mouth.

If you get distracted, do not try to change it or be hard on yourself about it.

Notice what you are thinking and keep focusing on your breathing.

After a few minutes, gently open your eyes and look around the room.

- **Example Practice 2: Body scan**

You can close your eyes if that feels comfortable for you.

Feel the contact of your body with the chair, the bed or the floor.

Notice your back wherever you are sitting or lying down. Take a breath.

Notice your hands. Are your hands tense or tight?

Notice your arms. Do you feel any sensation in your shoulders. Let them be soft.

Notice your legs. Continue to breathe.

Soften your face and then be aware of your whole body the best you can.

After a few minutes, when you are ready you can open your eyes.

Mindfulness practice could be introduced in shorter sessions using supported communication strategies with the addition of further adaptations (for example, visual prompts and audio tracks). A qualitative study (Jani, Simpson, Lawrence, Simpson, & Mercer, 2018) offered MBSR taster sessions to stroke survivors and it suggested that caregiver involvement could be a source of motivation and support.

People with aphasia can benefit from practical advice and modelling with experiential practices. The aim of an initial session can be to share core mindfulness skills by providing education and practice. For example, focusing on staying in the present moment, on non-judgemental observation of thoughts or feelings and on awareness of breathing or other body sensations. Additional factors are important to consider regarding the use of mindfulness including fatigue or lack of motivation to engage in further practice for developing these skills. This should be explored further with the individual as part of goal setting.

Acceptance and Commitment Therapy (ACT)

ACT aims to explore the concept of psychological flexibility, which refers to our capacity to respond adaptively to the challenges life presents and in a way that fits our values (LeJeune & Luoma, 2019). The emphasis of ACT on acceptance of distress and 'getting on with life' is particularly relevant in stroke as many survivors experience long-lasting physical, cognitive and psychological effects that may persist for years post-diagnosis.

Acceptance refers to the readiness to experience things that we cannot change, and it encourages carrying on rather than putting life on hold until a problem is 'fixed'. This can be a difficult concept to communicate verbally and does not mean that one should accept a painful or distressing experience. An important element of ACT is the use of examples and metaphors to illustrate this ongoing struggle and to create space from unwanted or distressing experiences. The '*Quicksand*' metaphor is an example that can be described visually and it refers to the struggle for control that can cause further emotional difficulties. For example, if you struggle when you get caught in quicksand, you sink; if you stop struggling, you float. This can be used to promote acceptance and an intention to pursue alternative ways of coping.

Commitment emphasizes the importance of behaving according to one's values. It highlights a person's own strong intention to lead the life they want by moving the focus away from any limitations. In the context of aphasia, the focus on doing what matters can support discussions about what values remain unaffected or changed post-stroke.

The 'Hexaflex' matrix (Figure 6.2) is central to ACT (Hayes, Luoma, Bond, Masuda, & Lillis, 2006) and it outlines its six core therapeutic processes:

1. Contact with the present moment: Connecting with what is happening in the 'here and now' including the practice of mindfulness skills.

2. Self as context: Developing the 'observing self' - we are not our thoughts, feelings or experienced sensations.

3. Cognitive defusion: The ability to notice your thoughts, sensations and feelings by being less caught up or pushed around by them.

4. Acceptance: Being human, allowing these internal experiences to be there and have that willingness that they will be there.

5. Values: The focus on doing what matters, identifying values that are personally relevant to the person.

6. Committed action: Purposeful engagement in activities and behaviours that are consistent with a person's values.

ACT delivered didactically to groups of stroke survivors proved feasible and

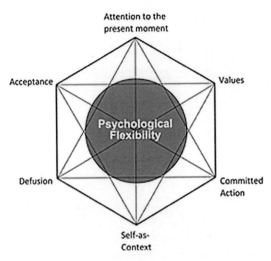

Figure 6.2 ACT 'Hexaflex' (Hayes et al., 2006). From Gilbert, *The Compassionate Mind* (2009), reprinted with permission from Little Brown Book Group. www.compassionatemind.co.uk

acceptable with benefits for depression and health status when compared to standard treatment (Majumdar & Morris, 2019). ACT appears to have potential as a psychological intervention for stroke survivors and its impact can be enhanced with certain adaptations in the delivery format (e.g., accessible easy-to-read handouts, regular breaks, limited distractions) (Large, Samuel, & Morris, 2020).

Goal setting is a key part of ACT and an effective way of engaging people with communication problems. It can be used to differentiate between values and goals with the aim to facilitate a bespoke and personal action plan during the rehabilitation process. ACT can be used to identify a person's value-based goals and to encourage committed action. The language used in this model encourages the person to lead a life that matters to them.

Illustrative example of values-based goal setting

Questions to consider for guiding a conversation about *committed action* based on a person's *values*:

- How would I like my life after stroke to improve?
- What would I like to achieve each day?

- If my life was a little bit better, how would that look like?

Break down into steps consistent with goal-setting and purposeful engagement:

- Identify the value: 'Maintain relationships with people in my life I care about'.

- Decide on a specific goal: 'Spend more time with my grandchildren'.

- Start with a small, realistic activity: 'Join them when they go out in the park'.

- Break down the goal into small, practical steps: Step 1) Find when they can visit; 2) Ask a family member to join and to help out; 3) Write the time and place for when they visit; 4) Arrange to do this once a month.

- Set a time for when the person could achieve or start the activity: 'I will aim go out with them within the next month. They are visiting this Sunday and I could talk to them about this.'

Morris et al.'s (2017a) book on rebuilding life after stroke includes further examples and visual illustrations on ACT-based exercises. This is available to borrow as an electronic free resource for people with aphasia at Reading Well booklists (https://reading-well.org.uk/books/books-on-prescription/16840135). Assessing the extent to how well the person can engage in talking therapies is essential. A key consideration with ACT-based interventions when working with people with aphasia is to apply them flexibly and consider whether it is appropriate to involve a family member in the process.

Suggested adaptations for using ACT

- Shorter and more frequent sessions.

- Repetition and slower pace presentation.

- Providing education to the core processes of ACT, e.g., values to support the identification of goals, committed action consistent with one's values.

- Simple and less abstract metaphors drawn from the person's personal experience. Freely available examples of metaphors can be found here: https://www.getselfhelp.co.uk/metaphors.htm, https://contextualscience.org/metaphors

- Shorter mindfulness exercises, consider the use of audio or video recordings.
- Using supported communication aids, e.g., pictures, values cards (adapted from Miller, C'de Baca, Matthews, & Wilbourne, 2001).

Compassion Focused Therapy

Compassion Focused Therapy (CFT) was developed by Professor Paul Gilbert (Gilbert, 2010a) for clients who experienced high levels of self-criticism, shame and depression. Professor Gilbert developed this therapeutic approach after years of working with people who had mental health difficulties. He observed that self-criticism and shame were significant barriers to progress in psychological therapy. Stroke, and in particular aphasia, can be highly shame activating, therefore a therapeutic approach which focuses on shame-based depression and anxiety may be helpful with this patient group.

The CFT model suggests that there are three emotional regulation systems (Gilbert, 2010b): the drive system, the threat system and the compassion system. The **drive system** is focused on achievement and pursuing goals. It is incentive- and resource-driven and creates focus and feelings of excitement/activation. The **threat system** is associated with safety seeking and protection. It tends to elicit feelings of anger, anxiety and fear. The threat system can be

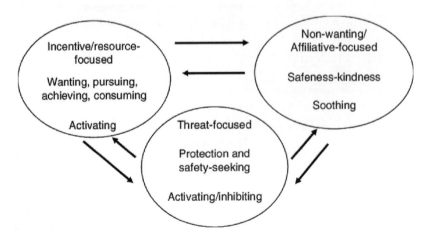

Figure 6.3 Emotional regulation systems: 3 circles model (by Paul Gilbert).

activating or inhibiting (fight or flight). Finally, the **compassion system** is centred on feeling safe, connected and soothed. It is the system that gives feelings of warmth and contentment.

Shame can present itself in a host of ways with individuals who have had a stroke, and for their families. For example, shame feelings can be activated by loss of bodily control, mobility problems, loss of role in the family or at work and the associated financial difficulties, changes in independence such as needing others to assist with daily care needs or not being able to drive. These significant changes in physical, cognitive, communication abilities, self-identity, changes in roles in relationships and work can trigger feelings of vulnerability and shame (Gilbert, 2015).

Shame can interact with rehabilitation and engagement with the multidisciplinary team in a number of overt and hidden ways. People may begin to disengage with therapy because they find it shaming and threatening to self-esteem. Think about how this might feel for a patient who has had a stroke; rehabilitation necessarily focuses on the things we struggle with and find difficult. Most of us have spent our adult lives avoiding looking and feeling incompetent or lacking in any way. We find areas of work and social lives where we feel competent and continue to develop these areas of our lives. Rehabilitation focuses on areas of our lives and abilities that we previously felt capable and competent in, but now experiencing difficulties can trigger feelings of shame. Stroke, and particularly aphasia, can limit an individual's ability to connect with others emotionally. Furthermore, they may feel they lack the time to focus on activities that give them a feeling of contentedness or safety as a result of rehabilitation demands and a focus on practical concerns which is typical in the early months of recovery post-stroke. Stroke is hugely threatening to the sense of self and identity; therefore, the threat system is activated, and for many people, the drive system and compassion systems feel diminished and hard to access. The CFT model suggests that psychological difficulties result from an imbalance between the systems which, as described above, can be common for people who have experienced a stroke (Ashworth, 2018).

The aims of CFT are to alleviate psychological distress associated with shame and self-criticism by using shame-reducing psychoeducation and helping patients to develop skills for self-soothing and self-compassion using Compassionate Mind Training (CMT). This is the most crucial part for patients with aphasia and their families as this training can be incorporated into their rehabilitation plan. The aim of this approach is to help people who have had a stroke to understand the need for balance in their emotional regulation systems. The three-legged stool analogy can be helpful in understanding this need for balance: if one is shorter or missing, the stool doesn't function well. CMT activities can be developed to focus on increasing self-soothing feelings. These activities include breathing exercises, compassion-focused images and mindfulness-based meditation skills, all of which can be adapted to people who have health and communication difficulties.

When working with people who have aphasia, it can be helpful to draw on experiences from their lives and knowledge from those close to them, to gain knowledge about activities which they may have found soothing in the past. Where you are uncertain, it can be useful to experiment with different options, tapping into activities such as colouring, music that is soothing, smells that bring a feeling of comfort, materials that stimulate soothing touch. Building up a compassion-focused image (Gilbert & Irons, 2004) can also be helpful; photographs or image searches can be used to activate the compassion-focused system and create balance. An excellent resource for freely accessible soothing images (Mok, Schwannauer, & Chan, 2020) has been compiled as a part of ProjectSoothe (http://www.projectsoothe. com) at the University of Edinburgh. Common themes for compassionate images include landscapes, trees and sky. For those who are able to access text reminders or alerts, this can be useful in initiating regular practice with the soothing/affiliative system. An alternative to this may be having visual cues such as a diagram of the emotional regulation systems or to use bean bags as a reminder of the need for balancing the three systems. These strategies can be used to support people to access their soothe system on a regular basis, outside of therapy sessions.

One of the helpful concepts in CFT is the terms 'tricky brain' as this can help to develop self-compassion and understanding that our brains are wired in particular ways that are not always helpful in the lives we are living. This is the case without a brain injury, but a stroke can make our already 'tricky brains' even trickier. This is not our fault, we did not choose this tricky brain that does not always serve us well, and we did not choose to have a stroke which made that even harder. Many of the ways we have developed psychologically, and the genetic predispositions to disease and ill health we have, are not our fault. This can help therapeutically as it reduces self-blame and guilt, which can be crucial in helping individuals integrate their experience of stroke and communication difficulties into the narrative of their lives and allow for a commitment to moving forward in a way that has value and meaning to them.

Conclusions

After many years of people with aphasia being excluded from studies assessing and evaluating therapies for psychological impacts, it is encouraging to see this changing. There are much-needed developments in this area, with current or recent studies including the feasibility of using motivational interviewing (Holland, Watkins, Boaden, & Lightbody, 2017), peer befriending (Hilari et al., 2021), solution focused brief therapy (Northcott et al., 2019; also see Chapter 3, this book) and early intervention by speech and language therapists for both the person with aphasia and their family (Ryan et al. 2017; Worrall et al., 2016). It is hoped that this momentum continues to build the evidence base for supporting and improving psychological wellbeing in people with aphasia.

References

Ashworth, F. (2018). Soothing the injured brain with a compassionate mind: Building the case for compassion focused therapy following acquired brain injury. In G. Yeates & G. Farrell (Eds.) *Eastern Influences on Neuropsychotherapy* (pp.77-120). London: Routledge.

Åström, M., Adolfsson, R., & Asplund, K. (1993). Major depression in stroke patients. A 3-year longitudinal study. *Stroke*, 24(7), 976-982.

Ayerbe, L., Ayis, S.A., Crichton, S., Wolfe, C.D., & Rudd, A.G. (2014). Natural history, predictors and associated outcomes of anxiety up to 10 years after stroke: The South London Stroke Register. *Age and Ageing*, 43(4), 542-547.

Ayerbe L., Ayis, S., Crichton, S., Wolfe, C.D., & Rudd, A.G. (2013). The natural history of depression up to 15 years after stroke: The South London Stroke Register. *Stroke*, 44(4), 1105-1110.

Baker, C., Worrall, L., Rose, M., Hudson, K., Ryan, B., & O'Byrne, L. (2018). A systematic review of rehabilitation interventions to prevent and treat depression in post-stroke aphasia. *Disability and Rehabilitation*, 40, 1870-1892.

Barrows, P.D. & Thomas, S.A. (2018) Assessment of mood in aphasia following stroke: Psychometric properties of the Dynamic Visual Analogue Mood Scales (D-VAMS). *Clinical Rehabilitation*, 32(1), 94-102.

Bennett, H.E., Thomas, S.A., Austen, R., Morris, A.M.S., & Lincoln, N B. (2006). Validation of screening measures for assessing mood in stroke patients. *British Journal of Clinical Psychology*, 45(3), 367-376.

Brumfitt, S. & Sheeran, P. (1999). *VASES: Visual Analogue Self-Esteem Scale*. Winslow Press Ltd. [Updated 2020, Guildford: J&R Press.]

Cuijpers, P., Berking, M., Andersson, G., Quigley, L., Kleiboer, A., & Dobson, K.S. (2013). A meta-analysis of cognitive-behavioural therapy for adult depression, alone and in comparison with other treatments. *Canadian Journal of Psychiatry*, 58(7), 76-85.

Dickinson, J., Friary, P., & McCann, C.M. (2016). The influence of mindfulness meditation on communication and anxiety: A case study of a person with aphasia, *Aphasiology*, 31(9), 1044-1058.

Eccles A., Morris R., & Kneebone, I. (2017). Psychometric properties of the Behavioural Outcomes of Anxiety questionnaire in stroke patients with aphasia. *Clinical Rehabilitation*, 31(3), 369-378.

Gilbert, P. (2010a). *Compassion Focused Therapy: Distinctive Features*. London: Routledge.

Gilbert, P. (Ed.). (2010b). Compassion focused therapy. *International Journal of Cognitive Therapy*, [special issue], 3, 95–210. doi:10.1521/ijct.2010.3.2.95

Gilbert, P. (2015). The evolution and social dynamics of compassion. *Social and Personality Psychology Compass*, 9(6), 239–254.

Gilbert, P., & Irons, C. (2004). A pilot exploration of the use of compassionate imagery in a group of self critical people. *Memory*, 12, 507–516.

Hackett, M.L. & Pickles, K. (2014). Part I: Frequency of depression after stroke: An updated systematic review and meta-analysis of observational studies. *International Journal of Stroke*, 9(8), 1017-1025.

Hayes, S., Luoma, J., Bond, F., Masuda, A., & Lillis, J. (2006). Acceptance and commitment therapy: Model, processes and outcomes. *Behaviour Research and Therapy*, 44, 1–25.

Hilari, K., Behn, N., James, K., Northcott, S., Marshall, J., Thomas, S., Simpson, A., Moss, B., Flood, C., McVicker, S., & Goldsmith, K. (2021). Supporting wellbeing through peer-befriending (SUPERB) for people with aphasia: A feasibility randomised controlled trial. *Clinical Rehabilitation*. doi: 10.1177/0269215521995671. [Epub ahead of print.]

Holland, E-J., Watkins, C.L., Boaden, E., & Lightbody, C.E. (2018). Fidelity to a motivational interviewing intervention for those with post-stroke aphasia: A small-scale feasibility study. *Topics in Stroke Rehabilitation*, 25, 54-60.

Jani, B.D., Simpson, R., Lawrence, M., Simpson, S., & Mercer, S.W. (2018). Acceptability of mindfulness from the perspective of stroke survivors and caregivers: A qualitative study. *Pilot & Feasibility Studies*, 4, 57.

Kauhanen, M.L., Korpelainen, J.T., Hiltunen, P., Määttä, R., Mononen, H., Brusin, E., Sotaniemi, K.A., & Myllylä, V.V. (2000). Aphasia, depression, and non-verbal cognitive impairment in ischaemic stroke. *Cerebrovascular Diseases*, 10(6), 455-461.

Knapp, P., Dunn-Roberts, A., Sahib, N., Cook, L., Astin, F., Kontou, E., & Thomas, S.A. (2020). Frequency of anxiety after stroke: An updated systematic review and meta-analysis of observational studies. *International Journal of Stroke*, 15(3), 244-255.

Kneebone, I.I. (2016). A framework to support cognitive behavior therapy for emotional disorder after stroke. *Cognitive and Behavioral Practice*, 23, 99-109.

Kontou, E., Thomas, S.A., & Lincoln, N.B., (2012). Psychometric properties of a revised version of the visual analog mood scales. *Clinical Rehabilitation*, 26(12), 1133-1140.

Large, R., Samuel, V., & Morris, R. (2020). A changed reality: Experience of an acceptance and commitment therapy (ACT) group after stroke. *Neuropsychological Rehabilitation*, 30(8), 1477-1496.

Lawrence, M., Booth, J., Mercer, S., & Crawford, E.A. (2013). Systematic review of the benefits of mindfulness-based interventions following transient ischemic attack and stroke. *International Journal of Stroke*, 8(6), 465–474.

LeJeune, J. & Luoma, J.B. (2019). *Values in Therapy: A Clinician's Guide to Helping Clients Explore Values, Increase Psychological Flexibility, and Live a More Meaningful Life.* Oakland, CA: Context Press.

Lewinsohn, P.M. (1974). A behavioural approach to depression. In R. Friedman & M. Katz (Eds), *The Psychology of Depression: Contemporary Theory and Research* (pp.157–78). Washington, D.C.: V.H. Winston & Sons.

Lincoln, N.B., Kneebone, I.I., Macniven, J.A.B., & Morris, R. (2012). *Psychological Management of Stroke.* Chichester: John Wiley & Sons.

Lincoln, N.B., Sutcliffe, L.M., & Unsworth, G. (2000). Validation of the Stroke Aphasic Depression Questionnaire (SADQ) for use with patients in hospital. *Clinical Neuropsychologist*, 1, 88–96.

Majumdar, S. & Morris, R. (2019). Brief group-based acceptance and commitment therapy for stroke survivors. *British Journal of Clinical Psychology*, 58, 70–90.

Mardula, J. & Vaughan, F.L. (2020). *Mindfulness and Stroke: A Personal Story of Managing Brain Injury.* London: Pavilion Publishing & Media Ltd.

Mazzucchelli, T., Kane, R., & Rees, C. (2009). Behavioral activation treatments for depression in adults: A meta-analysis and review. *Clinical Psychology Science and Practice*, 16(4), 383–411.

McLean, G., Lawrence, M., Simpson, R., & Mercer, S.W. (2017). Mindfulness-based stress reduction in Parkinson's disease: A systematic review. *BMC Neurology*, 17, 92.

Meredith, K.M. & Yeates, G.N. (2019). *Psychotherapy and Aphasia: Interventions for Emotional Wellbeing and Relationships.* London: Routledge.

Miller, W., & C'de Baca, J., Matthews, D.B., & Wilbourne, P. (2001). *Personal Values Card Sort Card.* New York: Guilford Press.

Mok, M.C.L., Schwannauer, M., & Chan, S.W.Y. (2020) Soothe ourselves in times of need: A qualitative exploration of how the feeling of 'soothe' is understood and experienced in everyday life. *Psychology and Psychotherapy: Theory, Research and Practice*, 93(3), 587–620.

Morris, R., Falck, M., Miles, T., Wilcox, J., & Fisher-Hicks, S. (2017a). *Rebuilding Your Life After Stroke: Positive Steps to Wellbeing.* London: Jessica Kingsley.

Morris, R., Eccles, A., Ryan, B., & Kneebone, I.I. (2017b). Prevalence of anxiety in people with aphasia after stroke. *Aphasiology*, 31(12), 1410–1415.

Northcott, S., Simpson, A., Thomas, S., Hirani, S.P., Flood, C., & Hilari, K. (2019). SOlution Focused brief therapy In post-stroke Aphasia (SOFIA Trial): Protocol for a feasibility randomised controlled trial. *AMRC Open Research*, 1(11). doi: https://doi.org/10.12688/amrcopenres.12873.2

Oates, L.L., Moghaddam, N., Evangelou, N., & das Nair, R. (2020). Behavioural activation treatment for depression in individuals with neurological conditions: A systematic review. *Clinical Rehabilitation*, 34(3), 310–319.

Orenstein, E., Basilakos, A., & Marshall, R.S. (2012). Effects of mindfulness meditation on three individuals with aphasia. *International Journal of Language and Communication Disorders*, 46(6), 673–684.

Panda, S., Whitworth, A., Hersh, D., & Biedermann, B. (2020) "Giving yourself some breathing room…": An exploration of group meditation for people with aphasia. *Aphasiology*. doi: 10.1080/02687038.2020.1819956

Richards, D.A., Ekers, D., McMillan, D., Taylor, R.S., Byford, S., Warren, F.C., Barrett, B., Farrand, P.A., Gilbody, S., Kuyken, W., O'Mahen, H., Watkins, E.R., Wright, K.A., Hollon, S.D., Reed, N., Rhodes, S., Fletcher, E., &, Finning, K. (2016). Cost and Outcome of Behavioural Activation versus Cognitive Behavioural Therapy for Depression (COBRA): A randomised, controlled, non-inferiority trial. *Lancet*, 388, 871–880.

Royal College of Physicians (2016). *National Clinical Guideline for Stroke*, 5th ed. London: Royal College of Physicians.

Ryan, B., Hudson, K., Worrall, L., Simmons-Mackie, N., Thomas, E., Finch, E., Clark, K., & Lethlean, J. (2017). The Aphasia Action, Success, and Knowledge Programme: Results from an Australian Phase I Trial of a Speech-Pathology-led intervention for people with aphasia early post stroke. *Brain Impairment*, 18(3), 284–298.

Scogin, F., Welsh, D., Hanson, A., Stump, J., & Coates, A. (2005). Evidence-based psychotherapies for depression in older adults. *Journal of Consulting and Clinical Psychology*, 12(3), 222–237.

Simpson, R., Booth, J., Lawrence, M., Byrne, S., Mair, F., & Mercer, S. (2014). Mindfulness based interventions in multiple sclerosis – a systematic review. *BMC Neurology*, 14, 15.

Stern, R.A. (1997). *Visual Analog Mood Scales Professional Manual*. Lutz, FL: Psychological Assessment Resources.

Stroke Association (2019). *Lived Experience of Stroke*. https://www.stroke.org.uk/lived-experience-of-stroke-report (Last accessed 26/04/2021).

Sutcliffe, L.M. & Lincoln, N.B. (1998). The assessment of depression in aphasic stroke patients: The development of the Stroke Aphasic Depression Questionnaire. *Clinical Rehabilitation*, 12(6), 506–513.

Thomas, S.A. & Lincoln, N.B. (2008). Predictors of emotional distress after stroke. *Stroke*, 39(4), 1240-1245.

Thomas, S.A., Walker, M.F., Macniven, J.A., Haworth, H., & Lincoln, N.B. (2013). Communication and Low Mood (CALM): A randomized controlled trial of behavioural therapy for stroke patients with aphasia. *Clinical Rehabilitation*, 27(5), 398–408.

Thomas, S.A., Drummond, A.E., Lincoln, N.B., Palmer, R.L., das Nair, R., Latimer, N.R., Hackney, G.L., Mandefield, L., Walters, S.J., Hatton, R.D., Cooper, C.L., Chater, T.F., England, T.J., Callaghan, P., Coates, E., Sutherland, K.E., Eshtan, S.J., & Topcu, G. (2019). Behavioural activation therapy for post-stroke depression: The BEADS feasibility RCT. *Health Technology Assessment*, 23(47), 1–176.

Townend, E., Brady, M., & McLaughlan, K. (2007). A systematic evaluation of the adaptation of depression diagnostic methods for stroke survivors who have aphasia. *Stroke*, 38(11), 3076-3083.

Turner-Stokes, L., Kalmus, M., Hirani, D., & Clegg, F. (2005). The Depression Intensity Scale Circles (DISCS): A first evaluation of a simple assessment tool for depression in the context of brain injury. *Journal of Neurology, Neurosurgery and Psychiatry*, 76(9), 1273–1278.

van Dijk, M.J., de Man-van Ginkel, J.M., Hafsteinsdóttir, T.B., & Schuurmans, M.J. (2016). Identifying depression post-stroke in patients with aphasia: A systematic review of the reliability, validity and feasibility of available instruments. *Clinical Rehabilitation*, 30(8), 795–810.

Wang, X., Smith, C., Ashley, L., & Hyland, M.E. (2019). Tailoring self-help mindfulness and relaxation techniques for stroke survivors: Examining preferences, feasibility and acceptability. *Frontiers in Psychology*, 10, 391.

Watkins, C., Leathley, M., Daniels, L., Dickinson, H., Lightbody, C.E., van den Broek, M., & Jack, C.I.A. (2001). The signs of depression scale in stroke: How useful are nurses' observations? *Clinical Rehabilitation*, 15, 456.

Wood, K., Lawrence, M., Jani, B., Simpson, R., & Mercer, SW. (2017). Mindfulness-based interventions in epilepsy: A systematic review. *BMC Neurology, 17*, 52.

Worrall, L., Ryan, B., Hudson, K., Kneebone, I., Simmons-Mackie, N., Khan, A., Hoffmann, T., Power, E., Togher, L., & Rose, M. (2016). Reducing the psychosocial impact of aphasia on mood and quality of life in people with aphasia and the impact of caregiving in family members through the Aphasia Action Success Knowledge (Aphasia ASK) program: Study protocol for a randomized controlled trial. *Trials*, 17, 153.

7 Living long-term with aphasia: The experience of the individual and their family

Dee Webster, Peter McGriskin and Carol McGriskin

Introduction

Aphasia is typically a chronic condition, affecting the conversations, relationships and lives of individuals and their families for many years post-stroke. This chapter seeks to explore and describe our understanding of living with aphasia in the longer term by individuals with aphasia and their family, and the implications for Speech and Language Therapy services.

We draw on the experiences and expertise of Peter, an individual living with aphasia, and his wife Carol. Peter and Carol are known to the first author through their involvement initially with Speech and Language Therapy services and latterly local aphasia voluntary organizations. Peter had two strokes in quick succession nine years ago resulting in aphasia, apraxia of speech and mobility difficulties. Prior to this, he worked full-time as a director of a large multinational organization. Carol worked as a teacher prior to Peter's stroke.

The content of this chapter has been co-developed through a series of conversations with Peter and Carol to discuss their experiences of living with aphasia. Supportive strategies were used to facilitate access to information and topics under discussion, with Peter using a range of techniques to convey his opinions and views. We considered carefully how to represent authentically the perspectives of all authors, particularly Peter as an individual with aphasia. Peter and the lead author discussed the importance of not overinterpreting his responses and we agreed on how we could represent his voice via a range of means. Where Peter's experience has been described in words, this is drawn from conversations with Peter expressing his ideas using a total communication approach and using a range of communication channels; the words used have then been reviewed with him to ensure that they represent his views accurately.

What do we know about the longer-term needs of individuals with aphasia and their families?

Adapting to life with aphasia is unique to each individual and family. Progress towards living well with aphasia, in whatever way this is personally defined, is an ongoing process. It is nonlinear, is complex, and is influenced by factors both internal and external to the individual and family (Brown, Worrall, Davidson, & Howe, 2012; Parr, Duchan, & Pound, 2003).

Despite the experience of living with aphasia being highly individual, some common themes can be found across research studies in this area. Wray and Clarke (2017) in their review of the qualitative literature, draw out four overarching themes in describing the process of adapting to life post-stroke by individuals with communication difficulties: communication with others and in particular managing communication outside of the home; creating a meaningful role; creating or maintaining a support network; and taking control and actively moving forward with life. Brown and colleagues also identify similar themes in the context of living successfully with aphasia: doing things; meaningful relationships; striving for a positive way of life; and communication (Brown, Worrall, Davidson, & Howe, 2010, 2011b, 2012).

We turn to these areas as we focus on the lived experience of those with aphasia and their families.

Communication with others

The importance of using strategies to support conversations with people with aphasia is well established (Kagan, 1998; Turner & Whitworth, 2006). Use of such techniques enables individuals to access and engage in meaningful conversations by working together to reveal communicative competence, build connection, and in turn develop and maintain relationships, with a view to enabling access to daily activities and increasing social participation. Use of supportive strategies can be targeted in Speech and Language Therapy effectively by working with the individual and their usual conversation partner(s) such as a family member or friend (Beeke et al., 2014; Best et al., 2016).

However, beyond the home environment, the sheer range of social situations and the subsequent skill and awareness on the part of potential conversation partners can be particularly challenging in providing the necessary ingredients for successful communication. Conversations in less familiar contexts can place the individual at increased risk of 'losing face'; Simmons-Mackie and

Damico (2007, p.92) describe the "delicate interactional and social balance between making meaning and saving face" for people with aphasia, and this is an important factor when we consider the acceptability of using supportive strategies within a range of different communicative contexts with a variety of communication partners.

Coupled with the lack of public awareness about aphasia, the lack of acceptance and awareness of alternative communication means, and the many barriers that exist at a community and societal level (Code, 2020; Simmons-Mackie et al.. 2020), the community landscape can be challenging to navigate with aphasia. This therefore can impact greatly on access to healthcare, leisure activities and general interactions outside of the home, and subsequently an increased need for family members to facilitate communication.

This is reflected in Peter and Carol's experience:

Here Peter shares some of the tools he uses to communicate. Picture 1 is his diary where he captures his activities using drawing alongside tickets and programmes from events and activities. He will sometimes refer to this during conversations with others. He also shares here (Picture 2) an example of using drawing from a conversation where he was expressing how he was feeling and what he was hoping to feel in the future. Peter describes using a range of 'tools'

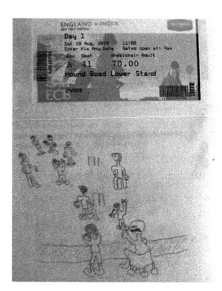
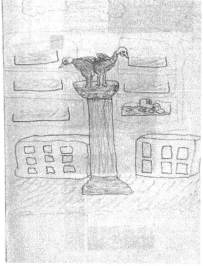

Picture 1.

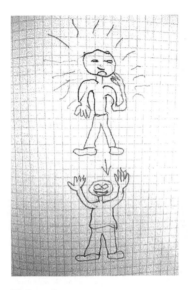

Picture 2.

during conversations including speaking, writing, gesture, facial expression, miming, and his iPad (using his calendar, the internet or photos for example).

Peter rated his satisfaction with conversations at home as 5/5 and those outside of the home as 2/5. He described using a range of techniques when at home, but that he is less likely to use these when out in the community, preferring for Carol to take the lead. Peter indicated that at home he felt he was more relaxed and felt comfortable using a range of tools. Outside of the home, he felt that others wouldn't understand, highlighting embarrassment about his communication. He expressed that using different ways of communicating would draw attention to him and he therefore often chooses not to be in this position.

> **Carol**: I see my role as a facilitator in helping Peter's communication and providing opportunities for him to speak with others. This is ongoing. I find relevant apps, develop aids to assist or practise speech, access local support groups and encourage him to take part in relevant research. I feel sometimes Peter tends to over-rely on me for cues and prompts to lead him into a word. He still wants to speak the word, even when struggling, rather than use strategies. We sometimes use visual prompts and we use lead-in sentences for everyday functional phrases.

Of course, for spouses and family members of those with aphasia, they too experience great change in their conversations within and beyond the home, with communication being described as the most difficult aspect of caring for a spouse with aphasia (Bakas, Kroenke, Plue, Perkins, & Williams, 2006). Carol describes the impact of stroke and aphasia on everyday conversations:

> **Carol**: In the early days, I don't think I realised how far-reaching Peter's aphasia would be, and how it would impact him and the family. There's an aching sense of loss, not only for personal conversations and debates about politics or events in the world, but for the minutiae of everyday conversations: watching television, and at a crucial point asking him, 'What did she say?' Trying to remember a forgotten strand of a shared memory; involving Peter in a phone call with family; our sense of humour, revolving around a play on words. Now every conversation is stunted, stop, start, recap. It's the loss of fluidity and spontaneity. What's kept us both going is hope. Hope that in 2 years, 5 years, it'll get better; now, at 9 years, hope has been dented by the recent Covid-19 pandemic as it has with many people, lockdown and isolation; there's a feeling of 'What's the point?' creeping in, but we both know we cannot afford to lose hope, so have to re-build.

An evolving sense of identity and role(s)

Many individuals with aphasia describe its profound and abrupt effect on their sense of self, individual purpose, life roles, and relationship within and with the world. Shadden (2005) describes aphasia as "identity theft" and considers the way that aphasia enforces a renegotiation of the identity of both the individual and their significant other.

> **Carol and Peter**: Peter misses his job, the status it held; his ability to mentor and guide others in their careers. Even post-stroke, for many years he identified himself as a successful, but disabled man. I believe his retirement has compounded his feelings of loss. Latterly he has focused on his loss of identity, freedom and independence. Because of the stroke and aphasia, his freedom has been greatly reduced, so he's gone from a man who was a free spirit, travelling the world for business, to someone who relies on me to organise his life.

> Up until recently, Peter has coped and adapted well, but as time has gone

on (and likely exacerbated by the recent Covid-19 pandemic and resulting social isolation) he has become less proactive and has experienced lower mood and self-esteem. Soon after his stroke, he approached his stroke as a survivor, and was determined not to let his stroke beat him. Whenever he had a low day, we could go out for a meal, or to the cinema, and it would lift his spirits. I feel I'm grieving again; back at the time of his stroke, I grieved for the loss of our life hit by stroke and how it affected each one of the family, but we built a new-normal and worked together as a team. In the past year I grieved for my husband's fighting spirit, that is so much of him. There was a time, I could raise his spirits with a motivational talk – now it's a bit more difficult. As life begins to get back to normal, we hope to start rebuilding his confidence and self-esteem. It's a constant search for new ideas and projects to boost him. What neither of us can afford to lose is hope!

Our identity, who and what we are, is an evolving state across our lifetime. Our interactions and conversations with others mediate our relationships and shape and reveal our identity. It is clear from Peter and Carol's experience that a reduction in our opportunity for social opportunities (due both to aphasia and then compounded by the recent Covid-19 pandemic resulting in greater social restrictions) can greatly influence how we see ourselves and our place in the world.

Communication breakdown or lack of access to conversation can "[carry] the message of inferiority and devaluation by society" (Shadden, 2005, p.215); for individuals with aphasia it can mask who a person is, their skills, expertise, passions and opinions. Aphasia and its sudden and dramatic impact on language and communication thus compels the individual and their family to rethink and reframe all preconceptions about the present and hopes for the future whilst also processing and grieving the loss of identity and 'what might have been'.

The role of the spouse or family member of an individual with aphasia is affected phenomenally, with individuals taking on many more responsibilities and roles within the context of reduced long-term support and increased emotional and psychological burden (Le Dorze & Signori, 2010; McGurk & Kneebone, 2013; Winkler, Bedford, Northcott, & Hilari, 2014) in addition to new challenges specifically related to communication including facilitating and advocating on the part of their family member with aphasia and maintaining relationships within the context of compromised conversation (Brown et al., 2011b ; Michallet, Tétreault, & Le Dorze, 2003).

Kniepman and Cupler (2014) describe the nature of occupational change of spouses of individuals with aphasia post-stroke. They describe themes including a reduction or loss in social activities, a need to find a new 'equilibrium', a lack of choice, and a sense of ongoing uncertainty. In their work in this area, Grawburg, Howe, Worrall and Scarinci (2013, 2014) describe "third party disability", the significant negative impact on the individual as a result of their family member's health condition (in this case aphasia) and the specific effects on the health, wellbeing, activity and participation of family members.

> **Carol**: I feel that my identity has not changed as much. Life as a teacher meant I have always helped and supported others, always problem-solving; Peter's job meant we moved often, and away from family, so never had their support when the children were younger. I have always had to be self-reliant, so becoming a carer has maximised on those roles.
>
> I do feel a huge sense of responsibility, in that if anything happens to me, I worry what will happen to Peter. It's that sense of responsibility that has driven me to push/encourage Peter to carry on – for example with physical exercise to keep as active as possible as he grows older. Our big driver has been to have a good a future as possible.
>
> I feel I have had to become more assertive. For example, I used to cringe when Peter would haggle, but now find myself taking on his role! Someone has to!

Individuals with aphasia, often with the support and advocacy of family members, are often required to work hard to reveal their identity to others, beyond the lens of living with aphasia and stroke. This is particularly challenging within the context of low public awareness of aphasia. Here Carol describes one example of how she supports Peter to share who he is with others:

> We have made a photo album telling My Story on Peter's iPad; it's made up of a series of photos showing Peter's family, friends, work, hobbies, travels. He is able to show this to people to show them he is more than a person with aphasia in a wheelchair – he has an interesting past … and will make an interesting, if different, future.

Meaningful relationships

Individuals with aphasia demonstrate reduced quality of life compared to those living with stroke without aphasia (Cruice, Hill, Worrall, & Hickson,

2010; Hilari, 2011; Hilari, Wiggins, Roy, Byng, & Smith, 2003). We know that individuals with aphasia are at greater risk of social exclusion than those without aphasia (Cruice, Worrall, & Hickson, 2006; Cruice, Worrall, Hickson, & Murison, 2003; Dalemans, De Witte, Beurskens, Van Den Heuvel, & Wade, 2010; Parr, 2007) and experience reduced social networks (Davidson, Howe, Worrall, Hickson, & Togher, 2008; Fotiadou, Northcott, Chatzidaki, & Hilari, 2014; Northcott, Marshall, & Hilari, 2016) including a loss and/or change in friendships (Brown, Davidson, Worrall, & Howe, 2013). Influencing factors include a loss of work outside the home, a reduction or loss of friendships (sometimes due to a lack of understanding on behalf of friends or family about how best to support that individual), or difficulty in accessing social opportunities due to the additional consequences of stroke such as reduced mobility or ability to drive. Spouses and family members of people with aphasia also experience fewer opportunities to maintain and develop friendships (Michallet et al., 2003) which can also impact on their health and wellbeing.

Here, Peter and Carol's experience reflects these challenges and describes ways that they have forged new connections:

Here Peter describes his social network before aphasia (Picture 3) and now (Picture 4). He sees far fewer people now and although he has close family, they live some distance away and so opportunities for connection are infrequent. Peter describes that before his strokes, he had lots of opportunities for conversation, spending time with a range people at home and at work.

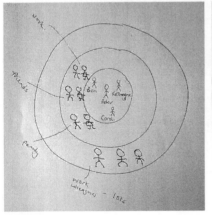

Picture 3.

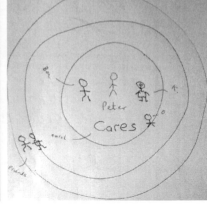

Picture 4.

Carol: Our children's relationships with Peter are affected and it saddens me to think what they've lost. They love him and are happy to see him, but he can't discuss the nuances of their careers, or advise them as he would want to. He'll never give the father's speech at their weddings, but he can still enjoy cricket and football matches with our son, something that is special to both of them.

Along with his loss of work is the loss of friendships – people who we thought were good friends have disappeared from our lives, maybe because they were embarrassed about how to approach Peter's aphasia, another who 'wanted to remember him as he was'! Others' embarrassment is nothing compared to what he is dealing with.

Although we've lost people we thought were close friends, we've made friends/acquaintances from across the world during our travels. Holidays and travelling were always important to us and we thought Peter's mobility would end our travels until we found cruising on small ships. We loved it, it gave us everything we thought we'd lost – good food and wine, dressing up, dancing and meeting new people – people who accepted Peter and his aphasia; people who didn't know him before his stroke; people who enjoyed our company, and we enjoyed their company. People from Australia, New Zealand, USA and Switzerland, who have kept in contact, invited us to their homes, and stayed with us in the UK. This is one aspect of our life we never could have imagined post-stroke, especially after losing friends to aphasia.

Finding others who have shared similar experiences can also be immensely valuable. Support groups for stroke and aphasia are becoming more commonplace and can act as a key source of ongoing support for individuals with aphasia and their families as well as providing a 'safe' environment to use a range of communication strategies.

Groups for people with aphasia are impactful in a range of ways. Attard and colleagues (Attard, Lanyon, Togher, & Rose, 2015) in their literature review of this area report that groups can support individuals with aphasia and their family members by: forming positive relations with others; supporting one another; finding purpose in life or 'giving back'; feeling empowered; and developing increased independence and autonomy, personal growth, and self-acceptance in living with aphasia. As well as providing opportunities for structured and more informal communication, groups can also serve as a bridge to attending other community-based activities.

Carol: We have also been involved with the development of a local self-help group for many years and enjoy social outings together. It's a good group of people, and while it caters for Peter socially, there are not always opportunities to develop and practise strategies as he is one of the few people in the group that rely on this approach.

It is good to meet others who have aphasia; it makes you feel less like you are on your own – that there are others living with the same condition. Seeing how others cope with aphasia can inspire and give hope and ideas to others.

The rise of virtual meetings recently has meant that we have been able to explore other groups, some with members around the country. They have weekly sessions to meet up and chat, giving Peter an opportunity to join in. He finds he's not embarrassed to speak or use his strategies among fellow people with aphasia.

As is evident, the content and approach of community aphasia groups needs to cater for the evolving and specific needs of individuals who represent a broad spectrum of aphasia severity. Groups need to carefully consider how to be facilitative to individuals with more severe aphasia (Attard, Loupis, Togher, & Rose, 2020) for the benefits of group membership to outweigh the costs to the individual.

One key finding in Attard et al.'s research is the importance of trying new, often creative, activities and the importance of this in finding meaning. The benefits of creative activities for people with aphasia have been explored, for example in relation to choir singing (Tamplin, Baker, Jones, Way, & Lee, 2013; Zumbansen et al., 2017) and photography (Levin et al., 2007) with reported benefits including increased wellbeing, greater sense of connectedness to others, and increased confidence.

Carol and Peter describe their experiences of exploring new activities:

Peter has been open to trying new activities, art, singing, adapted woodwork. We both attend an art group for people who have had a stroke. Peter had never had an interest in art, but we joined the group and both enjoyed it.

I am part of a choir and Peter comes to the regular end of term sessions. Music and dancing have always been important to us. He always joins in and is able to sing a lot of the words he'd be unable to speak spontaneously.

Peter also joined a woodwork group in a specialised workshop, with adapted tools. He made and painted a garden chair. This gave him a huge boost to his confidence, and was something neither of us could have imagined he could do, as he only has use of one hand.

For the past three years, Peter has also attended a brain injury support group once a week. This gives him an opportunity to meet others socially and chat, do creative activities and have some independence.

Starting with aphasia groups, we've 'dipped our toe in the water' and we have since approached a couple of community groups, e.g., the singing group, the village Petanque/boules group, and found people are mostly friendly and accommodating. This needs a degree of confidence from both of us, but we recognise that we're as much a part of the community as others.

Whilst groups can provide a valuable source of support for some people with otherwise limited access to social opportunities, they may not be the best fit for everyone. For those with aphasia who would find access to a group challenging, Conversation Partner schemes (McVicker, Parr, Pound, & Duchan, 2009) can also be of great value. Volunteers visit individuals with aphasia typically once per week and provide opportunities for conversation, interaction and a shared connection around a topic or activity of interest. Individuals with aphasia report a range of benefits, including opportunities to visit different community settings, opportunities to socialize, increased independence and increased confidence (McMenamin, Tierney & McFarlane, 2015).

Moving forward with life

The process of rebuilding life with aphasia and the ongoing nature of this takes a great deal of determination and energy on the part of both the individual with aphasia and close family. Readiness to try new activities or resume old ones also requires an acceptance of life with aphasia and a sense of self-efficacy, hope and belief in one's own ability to effect positive change (Bright, Kayes, McCann, & McPherson, 2013).

Carol and Peter: Fortunately, we both have a degree of bloody-mindedness, which has been essential in getting on with life. Stroke strikes everyone unexpectedly – there's no planning, one day you're getting on with life, taking it for granted, the next your world comes crashing down and you fear everything's ended. We decided we would not let stroke break us or our family.

It takes time, but slowly your battered confidence starts to emerge and you realise you still have choices to make a better future – you either let life happen, or you **make** life happen. We had always chosen the latter and our bloody-mindedness would keep us going forward and build the future we deserved.

The crunch moment came on our first cruise when we decided to get back in the game. We'd dressed for dinner; Peter in his evening suit, me in a stylish little number. We looked in the mirror, remembering all the black-tie dos we'd attended in the past, and said, "It'd be a waste to sit in a corner on our own, let's share a table with others." And we did. We sat with two couples, I introduced us, saying: "This is Peter, he's had a stroke. He's lost his speech, but not his understanding, or his love of red wine!" It wasn't planned, but it was an icebreaker, dispelling any thoughts that loss of speech may equate to loss of intelligence, and it was our first attempt to raise awareness of aphasia! As we approached the table, I still remember the stomach-churning moment of feeling I'd done something we'd regret, but it was a lovely evening, and we couldn't have asked for nicer people to help us re-enter life as we'd known it pre-stroke.

From that night, our confidence grew and we've sat at many shared tables, or we can have a table for two, but now we had a choice.

Recent restrictions in what we can do socially has taken away some of that confidence from both of us, but as life gets more back to normal, our bloody-mindedness will need to play a part again!

Moving forward also involves renegotiating your role within the world including work and professional role. Worrall et al. (2011) note that many individuals with aphasia hold "deep, strong desires to return to some employment", with a negative change in employment status frequently cited as an 'unmet need' in a survey of individuals post-stroke (McKevitt et al., 2011). Whilst this can be a key focus for Speech and Language intervention, very little is known from a research perspective about the experience of individuals with aphasia in returning to work and indeed the role that Speech and Language Therapy plays in this process.

For some individuals, the goal of returning to paid work may be realized, for others this need may be partially met by working outside of the home as a volunteer.

Peter has volunteered for a number of years as an advisor on a local aphasia advisory panel shaping Speech and Language Therapy services, and more recently as a Conversation Partner trainer. Peter rates being a volunteer as 'very enjoyable'. He expressed that he enjoyed the independence of doing something separate to Carol, finding out new information and learning from others. He also felt he was tapping into his previous work as a mentor, enjoying helping others and making a difference.

Carol describes volunteering at a local stroke research panel:

> We find it helpful to know what is going on in stroke research in order to increase our knowledge of stroke, hear about new ideas and also participate in research. We feel it's important to contribute to 'the greater good' and help other stroke survivors as well as adding to the scientific knowledge about stroke and aphasia.

The role of Speech and Language Therapy

Speech and Language Therapy tends to be delivered at its most intensive and frequent in the early weeks and months post-stroke, with access to therapy limited beyond one year (Palmer, Whitts, & Chater, 2018). Clinical and professional guidance does recognize the need for long-term support for individuals and their families post-stroke (e.g., RCP, 2016); however, despite this, access to therapy in the longer term is highly variable and is governed by local funding and commissioning arrangements.

Speech and Language Therapy services currently lack the resource capacity required to meet all the needs of individuals with aphasia (Code & Petheram, 2011), so resources need to be allocated carefully to optimize their impact on the life and experience of individuals with aphasia and their family members. Solutions can involve delivering therapy in creative ways, including group interventions and technologically supported approaches. It is, however, key that clinicians and service managers influence policymakers in order to ensure they understand the ongoing and long-term needs of individuals living with aphasia. Commissioners need to understand the value that specialist intervention provided by Speech and Language Therapy can have in addressing low mood, maintaining relationships, accessing community activities and services and improving overall health outcomes. It is by providing Speech and Language Therapy services which can flex and adapt to the needs of individuals with aphasia and their families that we can ensure that Speech and Language Therapy is available to individuals in the longer-term in a timely and impactful way.

Whilst a focus on ongoing language rehabilitation is a priority and can be beneficial for many individuals with aphasia, we know that the benefits of high quality, intensive language therapy can be limited in their impact on everyday functional communication and will not therefore fully meet the needs of people with aphasia. Indeed, goals focused on increasing activity and participation are reported as priorities for individuals with aphasia (Wallace et al., 2017; Worrall et al., 2011). It is recognized, therefore, that Speech and Language Therapy has a primary role in supporting individuals to live well with aphasia in the longer term beyond gains made at the impairment level, either as part of individual therapy or as a group approach (e.g., Armour, Brady, Sayyad, & Krieger, 2019; Mumby & Whitworth, 2012; van der Gaag et al., 2005).

A client-led approach with a focus on real-life communication, identity, connection, access to meaningful activities and a focus on wellbeing sits firmly within functional and social approaches to intervention encompassed by models such as the International Classification of Health, Functioning & Disability (ICF) (WHO, 2001) and Life Participation Approach to Aphasia (Chapey, 2008), incorporating the social model of disability (Mackay, 2003; Pound & Parr, 2017; Simmons-Mackie, 2001). In addition, recent work from Shiggins et al. (2020) has explored how the concept of salutogenesis can influence our clinical approach with people with aphasia and their families. This asset-based approach focuses on the opportunities, resources, community connections and perspectives of individuals with aphasia and their families rather than on deficit and loss. By re-framing our focus, Speech and Language Therapy can support individuals and their families to build on and reinforce these positive factors by working collaboratively with individuals and their families to find meaningful life experiences post-stroke.

Clinical intervention should be values-based: focused on the person with aphasia and their family as individuals with unique values and life priorities. Explicit focus should be placed on exploration of identity and supporting individuals to explore their sense of self within the context of aphasia and their individual circumstances and environments (Le Dorze, Salois-Bellerose, Alepins, Croteau, & Hallé, 2014; Simmons-Mackie & Elman, 2011; Taubner, Hallén, & Wengelin, 2020). Intervention should recognize the chronic nature of aphasia and evolving needs and circumstances of individuals (Grohn, Worrall, Simmons-Mackie, & Hudson 2014). This is supported by interviews with clinicians (Brown, Worrall, Davidson, & Howe, 2011a), yet a disconnect remains between this SLT perspective and the current service funding and provision for people with aphasia and their families.

Finding meaningful activities and roles

Opportunities for social participation should be explored with the client, including a discussion about how much social activity is actually desired. Each potential opportunity should be evaluated to see if it has the potential to align with the interests, priorities and evolving identity of the individual and establish what support might be needed to enable a positive, meaningful experience. In practice, this may involve signposting to local community aphasia groups, activity-specific groups, creating new opportunities, or intervention focused on specific community or leisure environments in order to maximize access and participation.

Some individuals may wish to take on a specific role such as group facilitator, educator or advisor. Self-help approaches to running aphasia groups can be particularly beneficial in enabling individuals with aphasia to explore a new role and find value in empowering others (Tregea & Brown, 2013). This can be meaningful for both individuals with aphasia and their family members. Some individuals with aphasia report the importance of altruism and being able to contribute to society (Worrall et al., 2011) and this certainly aligns with Carol and Peter's experience.

Connecting with others and building a support network

Given the risk of social exclusion for people with aphasia and the negative consequences of this, Speech and Language Therapy can play a key role in supporting individuals to maintain and find opportunities for meaningful social connection. This may be in the form of groups for people with aphasia and their families either face to face or online (e.g., Marshall et al., 2020), peer befriending schemes (Hilari et al., 2021), volunteering opportunities, conversation partner schemes, or in accessing leisure opportunities or hobbies.

Individuals should also be supported to navigate existing friendships as well as foster new ones. Azios et al. (2021) highlight the importance of clinical interventions that target the maintenance of current friendships. Published interventions focused on maintaining existing friendships are lacking; however, research from Davidson et al. (2008) supports intervention approaches targeting aphasia education, conversation strategies and supporting the individual with aphasia and their friend(s) to find meaningful connection through shared interests and activities, often using props, resources and supportive strategies creatively in order to access the humour, shared stories and connection found in conversations with friends.

Awareness-raising

Lack of public awareness of aphasia presents a significant barrier to community participation and integration for individuals with aphasia (Borsatto, Buchanan, & Pineault, 2021). In addition, this lack of awareness of aphasia and its impact on individuals and their families on the part of policymakers affects referral into, availability, and future funding of stroke and aphasia Speech and Language Therapy services (Simmons-Mackie et al., 2020). Whilst individual clinicians and services are often involved in campaigning to raise awareness of aphasia, the impact of such campaigns on public awareness has been limited. Simmons-Mackie et al. (2020) therefore suggest a targeted, collaborative, evidence-based, consistent international approach targeted to the specific audience (e.g., public, health professionals).

Managing endings

It is essential that clinicians work in partnership with individuals and their families in establishing when Speech and Language Therapy is required and when discharge is appropriate. Ideally, services should be structured to allow individuals to return to therapy at points when it is needed, empowering individuals to make judgements about their own health and wellbeing. Finding ways for individuals and their families living with aphasia to have ad hoc contact with Speech and Language Therapy services can be helpful in managing endings and discharge from services. Approaches might include links with local self-help groups, contact with individuals via communications such as newsletters, or drop-in sessions. Such long-arm approaches can ensure that individuals and their families are aware of any new initiatives or opportunities that may be of benefit in the future.

Conclusion

The impact of aphasia is far reaching and affects many aspects of the life of the individual with aphasia and their family members. Living with aphasia is complex, is highly individual and is influenced by the attitudes and values of the individual and family as well as external events and circumstances. Negotiating life with aphasia is an ongoing process and involves great shifts in identity, role and expectations, and changes in relationships and friendships. Individuals and their families describe the need to actively seek out opportunities for communication, connection with others, and finding ways of moving forward with life.

Speech and Language Therapy services must consider how they meet the needs of individuals with aphasia and their families in the longer term, shifting the focus of service provision to provide flexible, client-led and timely intervention with a focus on real-life communication, identity, connection, access to meaningful activities and a focus on wellbeing.

Speech and Language Therapists are also well placed to raise awareness of aphasia as part of a consistent, international approach to increase acceptance of total communication approaches and increase the likelihood of communication success for people with aphasia outside of the home.

It is by working alongside clients with aphasia and their families, gaining a clear understanding of their individual values, hopes and priorities from an asset-based perspective, that we can deliver effective, high-quality, relevant intervention and support individuals and their families to find meaningful life experiences within the context of living with aphasia.

Acknowledgements

With many thanks to Sally Knapp and Barbara Wilkinson for their insightful comments on earlier versions of this chapter.

References

Armour, M., Brady, S., Sayyad, A., & Krieger, R. (2019). Self-reported quality of life outcomes in aphasia using life participation approach values: 1-year outcomes. *Archives of Rehabilitation Research and Clinical Translation*, 1(3-4), 100025–100025.

Attard, M.C., Lanyon, L., Togher, L., & Rose, M.L. (2015). Consumer perspectives on community aphasia groups: A narrative literature review in the context of psychological well-being. *Aphasiology*, 29(8), 983–1019. https://doi.org/10.1080/02687038.2015.1016888

Attard, M.C., Loupis, Y., Togher, L., & Rose, M.L. (2020). Experiences of people with severe aphasia and spouses attending an Interdisciplinary Community Aphasia Group. *Disability and Rehabilitation*, 42(10), 1382–1396. https://doi.org/10.1080/09638288.2018.1526336

Azios, J.H., Strong, K.A., Archer, B., Douglas, N.F., Simmons-Mackie, N., & Worrall, L. (2021). Friendship matters: A research agenda for aphasia. *Aphasiology*, 1–20. https://doi.org/10.1080/02687038.2021.1873908

Bakas, T., Kroenke, K., Plue, L.D., Perkins, S.M., & Williams, L.S. (2006). Outcomes among family caregivers of aphasic versus non-aphasic stroke survivors. *Rehabilitation Nursing*, 31(1), 33-42.

Beeke, S., Johnson, F., Beckley, F., Heilemann, C., Edwards, S., Maxim, J., & Best, W. (2014). Enabling better conversations between a man with aphasia and his conversation partner: Incorporating writing into turn taking. *Research on Language and Social Interaction*, 47(3), 292–305.

Best, W., Maxim, J., Heilemann, C., Beckley, F., Johnson, F., Edwards, S.I., Howard, D. & Beeke, S. (2016). Conversation Therapy with people with aphasia and conversation partners using video feedback: A group and case series investigation of changes in interaction. *Frontiers in Human Neuroscience*, 10. doi: 10.3389/fnhum.2016.00562

Borsatto, J., Buchanan, L., & Pineault, L. (2021). Aphasia friendly Canada: The aphasia friendly business campaign. *Aphasiology*, 1–20. doi:10.1080/02687038.2020.1856328

Bright, F.A.S., Kayes, N.M., McCann, C.M., & McPherson, K.M. (2013). Hope in people with aphasia. *Aphasiology*, 27(1), 41–58.

Brown, K., Davidson, B., Worrall, L.E., & Howe, T. (2013). "Making a good time": The role of friendship in living successfully with aphasia. *International Journal of Speech-Language Pathology*, 15(2), 165–175.

Brown, K., Worrall, L.E., Davidson, B., & Howe, T. (2010). Snapshots of success: An insider perspective on living successfully with aphasia. *Aphasiology*, 24(10), 1267–1295. https://doi.org/10.1080/02687031003755429

Brown, K., Worrall, L.E., Davidson, B., & Howe, T. (2011a). Exploring speech-language pathologists' perspectives about living successfully with aphasia. *International Journal of Language & Communication Disorders*, 46(3), 300–311. https://doi.org/10.3109/13682822.2010.496762

Brown, K., Worrall, L., Davidson, B., & Howe, T. (2011b). Living successfully with aphasia: Family members share their views. *Topics in Stroke Rehabilitation*, 18(5), 536–548.

Brown, K., Worrall, L.E., Davidson, B., & Howe, T. (2012). Living successfully with aphasia: A qualitative meta-analysis of the perspectives of individuals with aphasia, family members, and speech-language pathologists. *International Journal of Speech-Language Pathology*, 14(2), 141–155.

Chapey, R. (Ed.). (2008). *Language Intervention Strategies in Aphasia and Related Neurogenic Communication Disorders*. Philadelphia: Wolters Kluwer Health/Lippincott Williams & Wilkins.

Code, C. (2020). The implications of public awareness and knowledge of aphasia around the world. *Annals of the Indian Academy of Neurology*, 23(Suppl 2), S95.

Code, C. & Petheram, B. (2011). Delivering for aphasia. *International Journal of Speech Language Pathology*, 13(1), 3–10.

Cruice, M., Hill, R., Worrall, L., & Hickson, L. (2010). Conceptualising quality of life for older people with aphasia. *Aphasiology*, 24(3), 327–347. doi:10.1080/02687030802565849

Cruice, M., Hill, R., Worrall, L., Hickson, L., & Murison, R. (2003). Finding a focus for quality of life with aphasia: Social and emotional health, and psychological wellbeing. *Aphasiology*, 17(4), 333–353.

Cruice, M., Worrall, L., & Hickson, L. (2006). Quantifying aphasic people's social lives in the context of non-aphasic peers. *Aphasiology*, 20, 1210–1225.

Dalemans, R.J.P., De Witte, L.C., Beurskens, A.J.H.M., Van Den Heuvel, W.J.A., Wade, D.T. (2010). An investigation into the social participation of stroke survivors with aphasia. *Disability and Rehabilitation*, 32(20), 1678-1685.

Davidson, B., Howe, T.J., Worrall, L., Hickson, L.M.H., & Togher, L. (2008). Social participation for older people with aphasia: The impact of communication disability on friendships. *Topics in Stroke Rehabilitation*, 15, 325–340.

Fotiadou, D., Northcott, S., Chatzidaki, A., & Hilari, K. (2014). Aphasia blog talk: How does stroke and aphasia affect a person's social relationships? *Aphasiology*, 28(11), 1281-1300.

Grawburg, M., Howe, T., Worrall, L., & Scarinci, N. (2013). Third-party disability in family members of people with aphasia: A systematic review. *Disability and Rehabilitation*, 35(16), 1324-1341.

Grawburg, M., Howe, T., Worrall, L., & Scarinci, N. (2014). Describing the impact of aphasia on close family members using the ICF framework. *Disability and Rehabilitation*, 36(14), 1184-1195.

Grohn, B., Worrall, L., Simmons-Mackie, N., & Hudson, K. (2014). Living successfully with aphasia during the first year post-stroke: A longitudinal qualitative study. *Aphasiology*, 28(12), 1405-1425.

Hilari, K. (2011). The impact of stroke: Are people with aphasia different to those without? *Disability and Rehabilitation*, 33(3), 211-218.

Hilari, K., Behn, N., James, K., Northcott, S., Marshall, J., Thomas, S., Simpson, A., Moss, B., Flood, C., McVicker, S., & Goldsmith, K. (2021). Supporting wellbeing through peer-befriending (SUPERB) for people with aphasia: A feasibility randomised controlled trial. *Clinical Rehabilitation*, 269215521995671–269215521995671. https://doi.org/10.1177/0269215521995671.

Hilari, K., Wiggins, R., Roy, P., Byng, S., & Smith, S. (2003). Predictors of health-related quality of life (HRQL) in people with chronic aphasia. *Aphasiology*, 17(4), 365-381.

Intercollegiate Stroke Working Party. (2016). *National Clinical Guideline for Stroke*, 5th ed. London: Royal College of Physicians.

Kagan, A. (1998). Supported conversation for adults with aphasia: Methods and resources for training conversation partners. *Aphasiology*, 12(9), 816-830.

Kniepmann K. & Cupler M.H. (2014). Occupational changes in caregivers for spouses with stroke and aphasia. *British Journal of Occupational Therapy*, 77(1), 10–18.

Le Dorze, G. & Signori, F-H. (2010). Needs, barriers and facilitators experienced by spouses of people with aphasia. *Disability and Rehabilitation*, 32(13), 1073-1087.

Le Dorze, G., Salois-Bellerose, E., Alepins, M., Croteau, C., & Hallé, M.-C. (2014). A description of the personal and environmental determinants of participation several years post-stroke according to the views of people who have aphasia. *Aphasiology*, 28(4), 421v439.

Levin, T., Scott, B.M., Borders, B., Hart, K., Lee, J., & Decanini, A. (2007). Aphasia talks: Photography as a means of communication, self-expression, and empowerment in persons with aphasia. *Topics in Stroke Rehabilitation*, 14(1), 72–84. https://doi.org/10.1310/tsr1401-72Liotta

Mackay, R. (2003). 'Tell them who I was': The social construction of aphasia. *Disability & Society*, 18(6), 811–826.

Marshall, J., Devane, N., Talbot, R., Caute, A., Cruice, M., Hilari, K., MacKenzie, G., Maguire, K., Patel, A., Roper, A., & Wilson, S. (2020). A randomised trial of social support group intervention for people with aphasia: A novel application of virtual reality. *PLosONE* 15(9). doi: 10.1371/journal.pone.0239715

McGurk, R. & Kneebone, I.I. (2013). The problems faced by informal carers to people with aphasia after stroke: A literature review. *Aphasiology*, 27(7), 765–783. https://doi.org/10.1080/02687038.2013.772292

McKevitt, C., Fudge, N.E., Redfern, J.M., Sheldenkar, A.D., Crichton, S., Rudd, A., Forster, A., Young, J., Nazareth, I., Silver, L., Rothwell, P., & Wolfe, C. (2011). Self-reported long-term needs after stroke. *Stroke: A Journal of Cerebral Circulation*, 42(5), 1398–1403.

McMenamin, R., Tierney, E., & MacFarlane, A. (2015). Addressing the long-term impacts of aphasia: How far does the Conversation Partner Programme go? *Aphasiology*, 29(8), 889–913.

McVicker, S., Parr, S., Pound, C., & Duchan, J. (2009). The Communication Partner Scheme: A project to develop long-term, low-cost access to conversation for people living with aphasia. *Aphasiology*, 23(1), 52–71. https://doi.org/10.1080/02687030701688783

Michallet, B., Tétreault, S., & Le Dorze, G. (2003). The consequences of severe aphasia on the spouses of aphasic people: A description of the adaptation process. *Aphasiology*, 17(9), 835–859.

Mumby, K. & Whitworth, A. (2012). Evaluating the effectiveness of intervention in long-term aphasia post-stroke: The experience from CHANT (Communication Hub for Aphasia in North Tyneside). *International Journal of Language and Communication Disorders*, 47(4), 398–412.

Northcott, S., Marshall, J., & Hilari, K. (2016). What factors predict who will have a strong social network following a stroke? *Journal of Speech, Language, and Hearing Research*, 59(4), 772–783. https://doi.org/10.1044/2016_JSLHR-L-15-0201

Palmer, R., Witts, H., & Chater, T. (2018). What speech and language therapy do community dwelling stroke survivors with aphasia receive in the UK? *PloS One*, 13(7), e0200096.

Parr, S. (2007). Living with severe aphasia: Tracking social exclusion. *Aphasiology*, 21 (1), 98–123.

Pound, C. & Parr, S. (2017). *Beyond Aphasia: Therapies for Living with Communication Disability*. London: Routledge.

Parr, S., Duchan, J., & Pound, C. (2003). *Aphasia Inside Out: Reflections on Communication Disability*. Oxford: Oxford University Press.

Shadden, B. (2005). Aphasia as identity theft: Theory and practice. *Aphasiology*, 19(3–5), 211–223. https://doi.org/10.1080/02687930444000697

Shiggins, C., Soskolne, V., Olenik, D., Pearl, G., Haaland-Johansen, L., Isaksen, J., Jagoe, C., McMenamin, R., & Horton, S. (2020). Towards an asset-based approach to promoting and sustaining well-being for people with aphasia and their families: An international exploratory study. *Aphasiology*, 34(1), 70–101. https://doi.org/10.1080/02687038.201 8.1548690

Simmons-Mackie, N. (2001). Social approaches in clinical practice: Examining clinical assumptions. *Advances in Speech Language Pathology*, 3(1), 47–50.

Simmons-Mackie, N. & Damico, J. (2007). Access and social inclusion in aphasia: Interactional principles and applications. *Aphasiology*, 21(1), 81–97. https://doi. org/10.1080/02687030600798311

Simmons-Mackie, N. & Elman, R.J. (2011). Negotiation of identity in group therapy for aphasia: The Aphasia Café. *International Journal of Language and Communication Disorders*, 46(3), 312–323.

Simmons-Mackie, N., Worrall, L., Shiggins, C., Isaksen, J., McMenamin, R., Rose, T., Guo, Y.E., & Wallace, S.J. (2020). Beyond the statistics: A research agenda in aphasia awareness. *Aphasiology*, 34(4), 458–471. https://doi.org/10.1080/02687038.2019.1702847

Tamplin, J., Baker, F.A., Jones, B., Way, A., & Lee, S. (2013). "Stroke a Chord": The effect of singing in a community choir on mood and social engagement for people living with aphasia following a stroke. *Neuro Rehabilitation*, 32, 929–941.

Taubner, H., Hallén, M., & Wengelin, A. (2020). Still the same? – Self identity dilemmas when living with post-stroke aphasia in a digitalised society. *Aphasiology*, 34(3), 300–318. doi: 10.1080/02687038.2019.1594151

Tregea, S. & Brown, K. (2013). What makes a successful peer-led aphasia support group? *Aphasiology*, 27, 581–598.

Turner, S. & Whitworth, A. (2006). Review: Conversational Partner Training Programmes in aphasia: A review of key themes and participants' roles. *Aphasiology*, 20(6), 483–510.

van der Gaag, A., Smith, L., Davis, S., Moss, B., Cornelius, V., Laing, S., & Mowles, C. (2005). Therapy and support services for people with long-term stroke and aphasia and their relatives: A six-month follow-up study. *Clinical Rehabilitation*, 19, 372–380.

Wallace, S.J., Worrall, L., Rose, T., Le Dorze, G., Cruice, M., Isaksen, J., Pak Hin Kong, A., Simmons-Mackie, N., Scarinci, N., & Alary Gauvreau, C. (2017). Which outcomes are most important to people with aphasia and their families? An international nominal group technique study framed within the ICF. *Disability and Rehabilitation*, 39(14), 1364–1379.

Winkler, M., Bedford, V., Northcott, S., & Hilari, K. (2014). Aphasia blog talk: How does stroke and aphasia affect the carer and their relationship with the person with aphasia? *Aphasiology*, 28(11), 1301–1319. https://doi.org/10.1080/02687038.2014.928665

World Health Organization (2001). *ICF: International Classification of Functioning, Disability and Health*. Geneva: World Health Organization.

Worrall, L., Sherratt, S., Rogers, P., Howe, T., Hersh, D., Ferguson, A., & Davidson, B. (2011). What people with aphasia want: Their goals according to the ICF. *Aphasiology*, 25(3), 309–322.

Wray, F. & Clarke, D. (2017). Longer-term needs of stroke survivors with communication difficulties living in the community: A systematic review and thematic synthesis of qualitative studies. *BMJ Open*, 7(10), e017944–e017944. https://doi.org/10.1136/bmjopen-2017-017944

Zumbansen, A., Peretz, I., Anglade, C., Bilodeau, J., Généreux, S., Hubert, M., & Hébert, S. (2017). Effect of choir activity in the rehabilitation of aphasia: A blind, randomised, controlled pilot study. *Aphasiology*, 31(8), 879–900.

Index